Early Detection of
Occupational Diseases

World Health Organization, Geneva, 1986

ISBN 92 4 154211 X

TYPESET IN INDIA
PRINTED IN SINGAPORE

85/6514 – Macmillan/Singapore Nat. Printers – 5000

Contents

CLINICAL AND LABORATORY TESTS FOR THE EARLY DETECTION
OF OCCUPATIONAL DISEASES IN THE MAIN ORGANS AND
SYSTEMS

ENVIRONMENTAL ASSESSMENT AND BIOLOGICAL MONITORING

Contents

Preface

An important aspect of the control of occupational disease is early detection, so that treatment can be given while the disease is still reversible. In 1974, the Executive Board of the World Health Organization requested the Director-General to undertake ". . . the collation and evaluation of methods for the early detection of health impairment in the gainfully employed . . .".[1] Early detection of occupational diseases was further emphasized in the Programme of Action on Workers' Health which was endorsed by the World Health Assembly in 1980.

As a step towards improving workers' health, this book has been produced as a guide for health professionals to the early detection of occupational diseases. The diseases included here are classified according to the hazardous substances that cause them and correspond with the list of occupational diseases adopted by the International Labour Conference at its sixty-sixth session in 1980. The book also includes chapters on the physiology of the main organ systems affected by the various chemical, physical and biological substances encountered in occupational settings and the tests that may be used for early detection of disease. The information presented in this publication is based on research carried out by WHO Collaborating Centres in more than thirty countries.

The final preparation of this book was done by a WHO Scientific Group on the Early Detection of Occupational Diseases which met in Geneva from 26 October to 1 November 1982. The Scientific Group examined, reviewed, and adapted material contributed by various authors specifically for the book. The contributors, and the members of the Scientific Group are listed in Annex 2. The World Health Organization is grateful to all those who participated in the preparation of this manual. Special thanks are due to Professor J. C. McDonald, who actively participated in the development of the publication from its early stages to the final draft.

Dr J. V. Homewood, Dr L. Ivanova-Čemišanska, Dr H. Thiele, and Dr E. Zschunke contributed papers on health education, the reproductive system, health examinations, and skin diseases, respectively. Information from these papers was used in the preparation of the book. The World Health Organization and the Scientific Group extend their special thanks to them.

---

[1] *Handbook of Resolutions and Decisions of the World Health Assembly and the Executive Board.* Volume II. Geneva, World Health Organization, 1979 (resolution EB53/23).

Introduction

Occupational diseases are caused by exposure to harmful chemical and biological agents and physical hazards at the workplace. Although they may appear to occur less frequently than other major disabling diseases, there is evidence that they affect a considerable number of people, particularly in rapidly industrializing countries. In many cases, occupational diseases are severe, and disabling. However, two factors make them easily preventable: first, the causal agents of these diseases can be identified, measured, and controlled; second, the populations at risk are usually easily accessible and can be regularly supervised and treated. Furthermore, the initial changes are often reversible if treated promptly. The early detection of occupational diseases is consequently of prime importance.

This book is intended to serve as a guide to the early recognition, diagnosis, and treatment of occupational diseases. It is addressed to health professionals at various levels responsible for occupational health. It is also anticipated that it will facilitate the organization of occupational health services at the workplace.

An additional function of this book is to create awareness among policy-makers, employers, and workers and their representatives of the possibility of preventing occupational diseases and of the preventive measures that should be taken by the occupational health services. It will also help countries in carrying out effective health monitoring of working populations and in obtaining adequate information on occupational exposure and its adverse effects on health.

At the present time, occupational diseases are under-reported and it is hoped that this book will encourage governments to adopt appropriate regulations concerning the notification of occupational diseases. It is recommended that regulations concerning occupational health should provide that every worker, if potentially exposed to an occupational hazard, should have access to health supervision and advice on appropriate placement and job selection from the medical point of view. All health examinations should be carried out during working hours and should be free of charge.

This book is divided into four parts. The first part (Chapter 1) deals with the principles of early detection of occupational diseases. The second part (Chapters 2–29) describes various occupational diseases and discusses approaches for their early detection and control. Chapters 30–36, which constitute the third part of the book, contain a discussion of the physiology of the body systems affected by occupational diseases, and describe clinical and laboratory tests for the early detection of those diseases. The final part of the book is made up of Chapters 37 and 38, which present biological and environmental methods for the assessment of exposure to occupational hazards. The occupational diseases discussed in the second part of the book correspond with the list of occupational diseases adopted by the International Labour Conference at its sixty-sixth session in 1980.[1]

---

[1] International Labour Conference, Sixty-sixth Session. *Amendment of the list of occupational diseases appended to the Employment Injury Benefits Convention, 1964 (No. 121).* Geneva, International Labour Office, 1980 (report VII(b)).

CHAPTER 1

Principles of early detection of occupational diseases

In 1973, the WHO Expert Committee on Environmental and Health Monitoring in Occupational Health[1] defined early detection of health impairment as "the detection of disturbances of homoeostatic and compensatory mechanisms while biochemical, morphological, and functional changes are still reversible". Thus, in order to prevent overt disease or disablement, the criteria of health impairment should, if possible, be based on the early biochemical, morphological, and functional changes that precede the occurrence of manifest signs and symptoms. One may distinguish the following broad overlapping categories of criteria of health impairment:

(*a*) *Biochemical and morphological changes that can be measured by laboratory analysis*—for example: disturbed porphyrin metabolism in exposure to lead; inhibited cholinesterase activity in exposure to organophosphorus pesticides; changes in the activities of various serum enzymes; changes in the concentrations of the components of body fluids; chromosomal aberrations; and abnormal sputum cytology. Some changes may be detectable only after loading tests, e.g., on excretory hepatic functions, or by other special tests.

(*b*) *Changes in the physical state and the function of body systems that can be evaluated by physical examination and by means of laboratory examination*—for example, electrocardiograms, tests of physical working capacity and, tests of higher nervous functions.

(*c*) *Changes in general wellbeing that can be evaluated by medical history and by the use of questionnaires*—for example, drowsiness and irritation of mucosa following exposure to organic solvents.

Health monitoring for the prevention of occupational diseases

The working environment frequently contains a wide variety of chemical, physical, biological, and psychosocial health hazards. The detection and assessment of occupational hazards fall under the discipline of occupational hygiene. This book briefly describes the methods of biological and environmental assessment, but it does

---

[1] WHO Technical Report Series, No. 535, 1973.

1

not deal with the principles of occupational hygiene *per se*. In any case, occupational hygiene alone is not sufficient to protect workers against occupational diseases; medical intervention in the form of preplacement and periodic health examinations is essential in the early detection and management of occupational diseases.

In all occupations, health examinations are designed to ensure that the worker is fit for employment and that he remains in that state of fitness throughout his period of employment. Any deviations from good health must be detected early and managed appropriately. Health examinations of workers frequently reveal the existence of health hazards in workplaces, thus necessitating environmental evaluation and control. Furthermore, they have important epidemiological significance in regard to such evaluation.

The appropriate preplacement and periodic medical examinations of workers as well as specific tests for the identification of early changes are described briefly below.

Preplacement health examination

This examination is carried out before employment and/or placement of a worker in a workplace with potential health hazards. The information it provides enables the doctor (and the management) to know the state of health of the employee, and the baseline data obtained are invaluable for follow-up of the worker in subsequent years. The examination also enables the management to place workers in jobs suited to their capacities and limitations. The medical information needed is recorded on a pre-employment examination form, the design of which varies with different occupations; often it contains a questionnaire on past medical, occupational, and social history.

Apart from a physical examination of various body organs and systems, the results of urine and blood analyses, radiological examination, eye examination, and, in certain cases, audiometric examination are included in the record. The preplacement health examinations should take account of individual risk factors such as age, sex, and individual susceptibility. Other influencing factors include nutrition, past or present disease states, and previous or concomitant exposure to one or more occupational health hazards.

Periodic health examination

The periodic examination should be carried out at regular intervals after the initial preplacement examination. It may not always be necessary to conduct a full-scale medical examination at the routine periodic check-ups, especially if there are no overt signs of illness.

The procedure for periodic health checks is different from that for preplacement examinations. A special form needs to be designed, with emphasis on the aspects of the history and physical examination most relevant to the exposure in question. The scope and periodicity of the health examination should depend on the nature and extent of the risk involved. The examination should focus on the body organs and systems most likely to be affected by the harmful agents in the workplace. For example, audiometry is the most important test for those working in a noisy environment. Workers in mines need radiological examinations of the chest to detect various forms of pneumoconiosis, and a clinical examination with special emphasis on the respiratory system. For each harmful agent, the period between exposure and the development of a health impairment (latency period) is a major factor in determining the frequency of examination. However, in many cases the latency period is not known. For such agents, the frequency should be determined on the basis of: (a) the natural history of the disease, including the rapidity with which the biochemical, morphological behavioural, etc. changes might occur or be detected by screening tests; (b) the level of exposure to the hazardous agent and to any other interacting agent or agents; (c) the anticipated susceptibility of the exposed population and individuals. Whenever possible, the manual recommends a frequency for periodic examinations.

Specific tests

Occupational exposure to dangerous materials, as well as the resulting health effects, can in many instances be evaluated by certain tests that are specific for the exposure in question. The analysis of biological material such as urine and blood can be used for the detection and evaluation of a chemical or its metabolite(s). The evaluation of lung function and X-ray changes in the case of dust exposure are often indicative of the degree of functional and pathological impairment. There are also other functional studies that can be used as specific tests for detecting the early, and probably reversible, stages of occupational diseases. These include electrocardiography, electroencephalography, evaluation of nerve conduction velocity, and audiometry.

The "normal" values obtained by tests on "healthy" individuals must be known in order to evaluate the significance of the values observed in exposed workers. The occupational health workers (including physicians and primary health care workers) should therefore know what should be considered "normal", preferably from data obtained by tests on workers that are not exposed to the health hazard in question or by comparing the findings in the exposed worker with values observed during tests carried out at the preplacement examination.

Specific tests should be selected in accordance with certain criteria, including validity, sensitivity, low cost, and safety. They are particularly valuable if they can be applied in the field by occupational health workers, semiskilled auxiliary personnel, and primary health care workers. Some examples of available practical tests are given below.

—For exposure to *organophosphorus pesticides*, a number of field kits for the measurement of total cholinesterase activity in blood are available.

—Where there is exposure to *dusts and organic fibres* (e.g., wood, jute, hemp), early impairment can be detected by tests of ventilatory capacity, e.g., vital capacity, forced expiratory volume in one second, and peak flow rate. These tests may be supplemented by a questionnaire.

—For evaluating the adverse health effects of *lead* exposure, simple, practical tests include the semiquantitative test for coproporphyrin in the urine.

—For the assessment of exposure to *trichloroethylene*, a simple semiquantitative method is available for the detection of trichloroacetic acid in urine.

—For exposure to *certain vapours and gases*, some field kits are available for measuring the agent in the air of workplaces. These can also be used for breath analysis (especially in the case of exposure to carbon monoxide).

—Routine blood count (haemoglobin, total and differential leukocyte counts) may indicate early impairment due to exposure to agents that affect *blood* and haematopoiesis.

—Routine analysis of urine for protein, urobilinogen, and bile pigments is indispensable in the examination of workers exposed to agents that may impair *renal* or *hepatic functions*.

Although the above examples indicate the existence of some practical tests, there is a great need to develop many more practical and simple procedures.

Need for workers' participation

In accordance with the principles of the primary health care approach, it is essential to secure the full participation of working populations in any health care programmes designed for their protection. This would not only ensure the efficacy of such measures, but also the continuity of a reasonable level of health at a low cost. In general, health and safety education and counselling are the commonly used means of securing workers' participation. Health education of workers aims to encourage them to adopt and sustain safe work practices, use working equipment properly, and make their own decisions (individually and collectively) to protect their health and to improve working conditions. The workers should be informed about the principles and practice of occupational health and the nature of potential health hazards in the workplace and should be encouraged to adopt practices that reduce health risks. Workers may be given health education either on the job (by workers' organizations, primary health care workers, or health personnel employed by the management) or during vocational training programmes.

Underserved working populations and primary health care

The majority of the working populations in the developing countries are underserved. Moreover, workers there are often economically disadvantaged, unorganized, and not protected by occupational health and safety regulations and labour protection measures; and their occupational health problems may receive little attention from the health services. In developing countries, the most important sectors in terms of occupational health are agriculture, small industries, and mines.

The most effective way of dealing with occupational health problems of underserved populations is through the primary health care approach. In occupational health, one may visualize the main functions of primary health workers as follows:

In rural areas, they would provide health care to the farmers who may be affected by the locally prevalent endemic diseases and malnutrition and, at the same time, be potentially exposed to the risk of occupational hazards, such as pesticides intoxication, work accidents, zoonotic diseases, and exposure to vegetable dusts, heat, and vibration. Thus, the primary health workers should have the ability: (a) to deal with general health problems; and (b) to detect certain specific health hazards and their effects.

Primary health workers may also deal with a group of small factories or industries in one area. They may undertake preliminary health surveys of these workplaces, collect environmental and biological samples and send them to specialized laboratories, identify potential sources of accidents and injuries, undertake first aid, maintain simple records, advise workers on safety and health matters, and refer sick workers for further medical care.

Intersectoral cooperation is essential for the success of preventive health care of workers. Industry, agriculture, labour and other social and economic development sectors must participate in workers' health services, particularly in the introduction of new technologies in developing countries since this often entails new health hazards.

Approaches to the early detection of the main occupational diseases

CHAPTER 2

Pneumoconioses caused by sclerogenous mineral dusts

Pneumoconioses caused by sclerogenous mineral dusts include: silicosis, anthracosilicosis, and asbestosis. Silicosis with pulmonary tuberculosis is also regarded as a dust-related pneumoconiosis, when silicosis is an essential factor in causing the resultant incapacity or death.

SILICOSIS, AND SILICOSIS WITH PULMONARY TUBERCULOSIS

Silicosis is a pneumoconiosis caused by the inhalation of crystalline particles of free silica (silicon dioxide). Silicosis with tuberculosis refers to the disease resulting from the interaction of silicosis with tuberculosis of the lungs.

Properties of the causal agents

The main crystalline mineral forms referred to as free silica (SiO_2) are quartz, tridymite, and cristobalite.

Occurrence and uses

Most rocks contain silica. Airborne particles of free silica are produced by blasting, grinding, crushing, drilling, and milling of rocks. Dusts from commercial workings of granite and sandstones and milling sand (silica flour) and heat-treated diatomite are particularly dangerous.

Occupations involving risk of silicosis

Workers in the following occupations are potentially exposed to the risk of silicosis: hard rock mining and extraction; civil engineering work with hard rock; stone dressing and polishing; casting, fettling, and sandblasting in foundries and in cleaning buildings; preparation and removal of refractory linings to furnaces, etc., and boiler scaling;

ceramic, porcelain and enamel manufacture; and the occupations in which sand is used as an abrasive.

Mechanism of action

Retention

The dust particles of 5–15 μm diameter deposited in the airways are cleared by mucociliary movement, but particles of 0.5–5 μm diameter landing in terminal airways or beyond may be retained. Most particles below 0.5 μm diameter remain suspended in the air and are breathed out (see Chapter 30).

The dust particles retained in the lungs are taken up by macrophages (mononuclear phagocytes) and transported either to the airways and cleared, or to the lung parenchyma. When the dust-containing cells die, other cells take up the released particles, but these too are killed, creating a continuous low-grade reaction leading to the formation of localized scars (nodules), which mostly occur around the terminal airways.

Free silica dusts vary in their ability to cause cell death, and this activity can be delayed by the presence of other dusts (e.g., oxides of iron and aluminium) and chemicals (e.g., polyvinylpyrrolidine N-oxide) that affect the surface of quartz particles. The normal protective mechanism of the body—coating dust particles with an iron-rich glycoprotein—seems to be ineffective in the case of free silica particles.

Elimination

The elimination of quartz particles, especially when mixed with other dusts, may occur in the first few days after inhalation via the bronchi and trachea. The percentage of the dust retained increases with: (a) increase in exposure levels; (b) higher past exposure to dust; and (c) the presence of lung diseases (especially tuberculosis). Particles retained in the lung parenchyma are seldom carried beyond the hilar lymph nodes. Therefore, the damage is confined to the lungs and the hilar lymph nodes.

Assessment of exposure

Environmental assessment

The best means of assessing exposure to crystalline silica in a workplace is by size-selective dust sampling in the breathing zone, preferably by using a personal sampler. Exposure may also be assessed by analysing respirable dust for crystalline silica content by X-ray or infrared radiation.

Biological assessment

There are no biochemical methods available for the assessment of exposure. Radiography can be used as a means of assessing exposure to free silica dusts. The radiographs should be interpreted using the ILO *International Classification of Radiographs of Pneumoconioses* (1980). The shadows seen on radiographs of lungs are caused by tissue reaction and not by the dust itself. At first, these are small, rounded and evenly distributed in all parts of the lungs, but later they may become irregular and coalesce, being then found especially in the upper zones of the lungs. However, because of the long latent period between the onset of the silicotic disease process in the lungs and the appearance and continued progression of shadows, the X-ray changes cannot be considered as an early indicator of exposure.

Lung function tests are also available for assessing exposure. Abnormalities in lung function coincide with radiological changes, though they are nonspecific and not useful as a measure of exposure.

The early stages of silicosis are symptomless.

Clinical effects

Silicosis

Acute silicosis is a rapidly progressive disease. In extreme conditions, breathlessness and dry cough may develop within a few weeks of exposure. Chest tightness and incapacity to work develop within months, and death due to respiratory failure or cor pulmonale may occur in 1–3 years. On examination, restricted chest movement, cyanosis, and late inspiratory rales are found, with restrictive lung function abnormality and reduced gas transfer. Radiography shows fluffy peripheral shadows that gradually harden to become linear. Often, these are not recognized even at autopsy because macrophage death and cellular reaction frequently occur in the alveoli without the formation of typical nodules. Doubly refractile silica particles are very numerous in lung tissue.

Under current working conditions, i.e., at levels of exposure normally prevailing in industrialized countries, silicosis develops only after many years of exposure. There is a wide variation in the rate of development and severity of disease, both of which depend on the level of exposure, the biological activity of the dust, and the presence or absence of substances that delay the tissue reaction. Initially, most of the dust is cleared. Later, with damage to hilar lymph nodes and lymphatics, the proportion of dust retained increases and the site of damage moves into the lung parenchyma. Whorled nodules of collagen tissue form around dust aggregations and constrict neighbouring blood vessels, lymphatics, and small airways, causing ischaemic damage to the lung and secondary scarring. This occurs most frequently in the upper and middle zones of the lungs and is seen on the X-ray as irregular shadowing with coalescence and calcification. The calcification of enlarged hilar nodes is also common.

The early stages of silicosis are as a rule not accompanied by any symptoms or signs of respiratory disease. Also, the basic ventilatory lung function tests remain within the normal physiological range. In more advanced stages, dyspnoea on exercise develops. Because of insidious onset, the dyspnoeic symptoms may be attributed to aging; X-rays are therefore a relatively more specific method of detection. The coalescence of shadows is accompanied by more rapidly progressive breathlessness during exercise and by depressed respiratory function, which is mainly restrictive in type. Bronchitic symptoms, e.g., cough and phlegm due to the deposition of larger dust particles in the airways are less important and sometimes reversible.

Silicosis with pulmonary tuberculosis

Workers exposed to silica are at an increased risk of tuberculosis, a risk that is substantially and permanently increased once X-ray changes are manifest. The infectious agent is usually *Mycobacterium tuberculosis*, but other types (e.g., *M. marinum* and *M. kansasii*) may also be responsible. The risk increases with severity of silicosis, and factors favourable for spreading tuberculosis include, for example, crowded working conditions, poor nutrition, and a high prevalence of infection in the community.

It is supposed that increased susceptibility of silicosis patients to lung tuberculosis is due to the damage caused by the dust to macrophages and to the lymphatic and immune systems, which normally protect against pulmonary tuberculosis. The suspicion of tuberculosis in silicosis should arise whenever there is a sudden increase in symptoms or X-ray changes, fever, loss of weight, or haemoptysis. The progression of X-ray changes continues to be more rapid even when the infection is controlled. The most reliable index of diagnosis or cure is the culture of mycobacteria in sputum; other indices are less reliable. Previous tuberculosis, treated or not, probably increases the risk and severity of silicosis.

There is no evidence of increased risk of cancer in exposure to silica dust or in patients with silicosis.

Exposure–effect relationships

Exposure to 1–2 mg quartz/m³ may cause detectable disease in 5–15 years, the X-ray changes starting first, followed by lung function abnormalities and the appearance of symptoms. At lower levels of exposure, there is a longer delay in the development of the disease, with symptoms often not appearing until after the exposure has ceased.

The exposure–effect relationship depends on: (*a*) the air concentration of the dust; (*b*) cumulative exposure dose (the sum of air concentration and duration of exposure); and (*c*) the "residence" time (the length of time the dust has been in the lungs). The frequency of the disease varies considerably from one industry to another, apparently independently of the level of exposure to free silica particles. It appears that exposure to low concentrations for a long period causes less severe disease than exposure to high concentrations for a short period. In the future, laboratory tests using cellular or animal models may be able to predict the risks from particular dusts more accurately.

Prognosis

The rate of progression of the disease is usually slow. It tends to slow down after exposure ceases, but symptoms increase when the coalescence of shadows starts. The final prognosis is difficult to predict until long after the cessation of exposure. Intercurrent respiratory infections and right heart failure are often the terminal events. Even when all exposure has ceased, the disease continues to progress, leading occasionally to respiratory failure or cor pulmonale in twice the time it takes for the early signs to develop. The results of antituberculosis treatment are considered, in general, to be less favourable when silicosis is also present.

Differential diagnosis

Characteristic early nodular radiological changes with upper-zone coalescence, lack of physical signs or much cough, and nonspecific lung function failure make the diagnosis of silicosis easy in dust-exposed groups. In individual cases, diagnosis depends on occupational history and on the exclusion of tuberculosis, lung cancer, sarcoidosis, rheumatoid arthritis, etc. by usual clinical and laboratory methods. The presence of complicating infections, such as tuberculosis, should be confirmed by sputum culture and appropriate serological tests.

Susceptibility

There is no evidence of differences in susceptibility between individuals. However, previous exposure to fibrogenic dust and the presence of tuberculosis increase susceptibility.

Health examinations

Preplacement examination

The preplacement health examination should include a medical history of the employee and a physical examination, with special emphasis on the respiratory system. A chest X-ray should be taken to see if the individual has pulmonary tuberculosis or any other lung disease. Basic lung function tests should be carried out, including measurement of the vital capacity (VC) and forced expiratory volume in 1 second ($FEV_{1.0}$).

Periodic examination

In medical terms the periodic examination is the same as the preplacement one. Its frequency depends on the level of dust exposure. If control measures are satisfactory, the examination could be repeated at three-year intervals. The objective of the examination is to prevent the emergence of disease during the working life of the worker. However, periodic examinations may not help in preventing the development of silicosis after retirement. Nevertheless, all X-rays, results of lung function tests, and data on individual cumulative exposures should be retained for epidemiological analyses.

If a significant number of workers develop silicosis within 20–25 years of first employment, the dust control measures at the workplace should be completely revised. It is also recommended that a medical examination should be done immediately if a worker develops chest symptoms, especially if tuberculosis is prevalent in the community.

Screening tests

Although chest radiography and simple tests of respiratory function (e.g., $FEV_{1.0}$), are of low specificity and late indicators of disease in individual cases, they are extremely valuable in monitoring exposure and disease when analysed for a large group of workers.

Case management

When the first signs of silicosis or active tuberculosis appear, the patient should be immediately withdrawn from further exposure. Although initially there is no need to restrict other work or activity, the patient should remain under continued medical surveillance. There is no treatment for silicosis. Treatment for respiratory or heart failure may be required in the later stages of silicosis.

It is important to prevent tuberculosis in silicosis patients. When the incidence of tuberculosis in the community is high, vaccination and chemoprophylaxis should be considered, although their value has not been proved with certainty. Tuberculosis patients should be treated early. Chemotherapy must be carefully supervised and should be appropriate for the prevalent strains of tuberculosis.

Control measures

The suppression of dust by technical control measures (pre-wetting, wet drilling, etc.) should be rigidly enforced and any residual dust should be controlled by proper ventilation. Respirable dust levels and free silica content of dust should be monitored regularly. Whenever explosives are used, workers should be prevented from entering the dusty area until the dust is cleared by ventilation. Dust should be filtered out of exhaust air.

Workers should wear masks, pressure hoods, etc. during breakdown of normal technical dust control measures or in emergency situations. Air-conditioned cabs should be provided for truck drivers and operators of excavators, cranes, etc. during open-cast operations in dry climates where water sprinkling is impossible.

There is no uniformity in exposure limits for silica dust in different countries. Exposure limits for total dust are mostly between 0.5 mg/m^3 (dust with high silica content—i.e., above 70%) and 5 mg/m^3 (dust with silica content less than 10%). For respirable dust the limits range from 0.1 mg/m^3 to 0.2 mg/m^3. The limits for cristobalite and tridymite are usually half of those for quartz.

ANTHRACOSILICOSIS [1]

Anthracosilicosis (coal-worker's pneumoconiosis) is a pneumoconiosis caused by exposure to mixed dust in which free silica is not the dominant fibrogenic component. In most situations, the relative importance of the components of the mixed dust in coal mines is not known.

Properties of the causal agent

Coal contains mostly carbon and some hydrogen, sulfur, and phosphorus, and a variety of rocks, some containing free silica. The composition varies from mine to mine and seam to seam. Mixed dust in coal mines may be derived from shale, oölite, millstone grit, kaolinite, slate, limestone, etc., all of which are frequently present within, above, and below coal seams. Coal itself may be the least important component of mineral dust.

Occurrence and uses

Mixed dust formed during coal-mining is most liable to accumulate in deep mines, especially where mechanical cutting of rock above and

---

[1] In *International nomenclature of diseases; volume III; diseases of the lower respiratory tract; 1st edition* (Geneva, Council for International Organizations of Medical Sciences, 1979), the term anthracosilicosis is included under silicosis.

below narrow seams occurs. Open-cast workings are less dependent on artificial ventilation. Once separated from rock, the distribution and use of coal creates less harmful dust. Along with oil, coal is the source of most of the world's energy and provides raw material for the chemical industry.

Occupations involving risk of anthracosilicosis

All workers in deep mines (especially those involved in development work and those heavily exposed in open-cast mines), workers in loading operations (e.g., on ships) and those in industries using coal (e.g., the steel industry) are at greatest risk of exposure.

Mechanism of action

Particles between 5 μm and 15 μm in diameter deposited in the airways cause reversible irritation (bronchitis). Most particles of 0.5–5.0 μm are cleared by scavenger cells via the bronchi and trachea, but heavy exposure leads to their retention in the lung tissue, lymphatics, and lymph nodes. Only if retention is very great (at least 50 g/lung) does low-grade tissue reaction lead to disturbance of lung function.

Assessment of exposure

Environmental assessment

Individual exposure can be assessed by size-selective dust sampling in the breathing zone, preferably by a personal sampler. Periodic analyses of bulk samples of respirable dust can also be carried out for component minerals.

Biological assessment

Biochemical tests. There are no biochemical tests available.

Radiography. This is the only available method of diagnosing anthracosilicosis. In the early stages of the disease, small, rounded, scattered shadows (opacities) appear on the radiograph. These do not increase with residence time. However, as the dust burden increases, the shadows enlarge, often leading to progressive massive fibrosis. The ILO *International Classification of Radiographs of Pneumoconioses* (1980) should be used in making the diagnosis.

Lung function tests. Lung function tests show no abnormalities in the early stages.

Symptoms and signs. Usually there are no signs or symptoms in the early stages.

Clinical effects

Clinical disease is preceded for many years by X-ray signs of simple pneumoconiosis, which by itself leads only to a slight acceleration in the normal rate of lung function deterioration. In most coal-workers, complicated pneumoconiosis develops only when the dust burden is very high. Reticulin and collagen deposit around large aggregates of dust, and this eventually leads to damage to blood vessels, airways, and lymphatics, with disturbance of lung function. The deterioration of lung function is associated with the formation of large rounded masses containing small amounts of collagen. This condition is known as progressive massive fibrosis. The rounded masses may undergo central necrosis and cavitate, rendering those areas susceptible to invasion by saprophytic microorganisms, particularly when antibiotics are used unwisely. There is no increased risk of tuberculosis, and there is no association between anthracosilicosis and lung cancer.

Exposure–effect relationship

Within a given coal-field there is usually a close exposure–response relationship between accumulated respirable dust exposure and the enlargement of small opacities on radiographs. Correlations between different coal-fields may not be very high. The amount of development work undertaken by miners probably increases the risk of anthracosilicosis.

Prognosis

If dust exposure is stopped at the early stage of simple pneumoconiosis (usually at < 2/2 p or q in the ILO *International Classification of Radiographs of Pneumoconioses*), little disabling disease occurs unless:
—the miner's work involves exposure to a high proportion of dust from mine development (rock) work away from the coal-face; and
—the worker develops rheumatoid disease with synergistic lung changes (Caplan syndrome).
In anthracosilicosis, serious disability occurs after exposure to much higher dust levels than is the case in silicosis. Furthermore, the disease is less likely to progress.

Differential diagnosis

An occupational history of prolonged heavy dust exposure in coal-mines coupled with typical X-ray changes and the relative lack of symptoms, signs, or loss of lung function indicate the presence of simple pneumoconiosis. In progressive massive fibrosis, there are clear-cut massive shadows on the X-ray, which are distinct from those seen in most other lung diseases (lung cancer, tuberculosis, sarcoidosis, etc.). The latter diseases can be excluded by appropriate investigations.

Susceptibility

Previous dust exposure and the presence of pulmonary tuberculosis or rheumatoid disease increase susceptibility.

Health examinations

Preplacement examination

The preplacement health examination should include a medical history, a physical examination with special emphasis on the respiratory system, a history of tuberculosis, and the presence of arthritis. A chest X-ray should be taken to see if the individual has pulmonary tuberculosis, and basic lung function tests ($FEV_{1.0}$ and VC) should be carried out.

Periodic examination

In medical terms the periodic examination is the same as the preplacement one. It is usually carried out once every three years. The results of periodic examinations provide evidence (clinical, radiographic, functional) for the epidemiological evaluation of exposure–effect relationship and help in assessing the adequacy of dust control measures. They also enable the management to identify workers with heavy dust burdens so that they can be transferred to jobs in which there is no dust exposure.

Case management

There is no specific treatment for anthracosilicosis. If characteristic X-ray changes of Caplan syndrome appear, the worker should be immediately withdrawn from work involving dust exposure, irrespective of the background X-ray changes. Workers with simple pneumoconiosis should also be withdrawn from work involving dust exposure. In both cases there is no need to restrict other work or activity.

Progressive massive fibrosis requires medical supervision and supportive therapy:

—for cardiac and respiratory failure;
—during episodes of melanoptysis resulting from the formation of cavities in the collagen-containing masses;
—for secondary infection of cavities;

—for spontaneous pneumothorax (this condition is common and should be treated conservatively).

Pulmonary surgery is not indicated in progressive massive fibrosis.

Control measures

The control measures recommended for silicosis also apply to anthracosilicosis (see page 15).

Exposure limits in most countries are related to the free silica content of coal-mine dust.

ASBESTOSIS AND RELATED DISEASES

Asbestosis is a progressive, irreversible silicatosis[1] caused by the inhalation of asbestos fibres.

Properties of the causal agents

Asbestos is a generic term for a group of naturally occurring fibrous mineral silicates. They are crystalline in form and are capable of splitting longitudinally into single fibrils or fibre bundles. Two groups and six mineral types are recognized: serpentine group—chrysotile; amphibole group—crocidolite, amosite, anthophyllite, tremolite, actinolite. All are chain hydrated silicates of magnesium, except crocidolite, which is a silicate of sodium and iron. Crocidolite and amosite have a large iron content. The amphiboles split into straight fibres of variable but mostly very narrow diameter (about 0.1 μm). Chrysotile occurs in sheets that curl up, producing hollow, tube-like fibrils of about 0.03 μm diameter. The properties that make asbestos unique are: relative insolubility, high tensile strength, and resistance to heat and acids (amphiboles only).

Uses

Asbestos has been commercially exploited since 1880. In 1979, the world production exceeded 50 million tonnes. In the same year 69 % of asbestos was used in making cement products, such as pipes and roofing sheets; 29 % was used to make other roofing materials, papers and felts, floor tiles, friction materials, paints and coatings; and 2 % was used in textiles, plastics, and insulation material. Asbestos paper, floor

---

[1] A general term for disorders arising from the inhalation of silicates with no free silica content.

coverings, and brake linings are mainly made from chrysotile. In other products, mixtures of chrysotile and amphiboles are generally used.

Occupations involving risk of asbestosis

Workers in the following occupations are at greatest risk of developing asbestosis: mining, milling, and processing of asbestos; transport of mined or milled asbestos; manufacture of asbestos products; disposal of waste material from asbestos mining, milling, etc.; any use or dismantling of asbestos products that causes airborne asbestos dust.

Mechanism of action

Inhaled airborne fibres of less than about 3 μm diameter penetrate the airways and are retained in the lungs. Since fibres of chrysotile are curly, they enter the lungs less easily than the amphiboles. A substantial proportion of the fibres entering the lungs is cleared from the respiratory tract in saliva and sputum. Of the fibres retained in the small airways and alveoli, some short fibres are engulfed by macrophages and carried to the lymph nodes, spleen, and other tissues. Some of the fibres that remain in the small airways and alveoli, (especially the amphiboles) are coated with an iron–protein complex and become "asbestos" or "ferruginous" bodies. It is thought that chrysotile gradually disappears from the body, but evidence of this is scanty.

After long or heavy exposure, there is substantial retention of asbestos fibres. This gradually leads to progressive, diffuse interstitial pulmonary fibrosis, with the individual acinar lesions gradually coalescing. Pleural fibrosis of variable degree is often found, and sometimes hyaline or calcified pleural plaques appear, which may not necessarily be asbestos-related.

Persons exposed to airborne dust swallow asbestos fibres with saliva or sputum. Sometimes water, drinks, or food may also contain small quantities of fibres. Some of the swallowed fibres probably penetrate the gut wall, but their subsequent migration in the body is unknown. After a latent period, rarely less than 20 years and up to 40 years or more after first occupational exposure, lung cancer, malignant mesothelioma of the pleura, or gastrointestinal cancer may develop.

The mechanisms of carcinogenesis are unknown. In the case of mesothelioma, animal experiments suggest that very fine fibres of about 0.1 μm diameter and a length of 8 μm or more are responsible. Mesotheliomas have rarely been reported after pure chrysotile exposure, but following exposure to crocidolite, amosite, or mixtures containing these minerals, mesotheliomas have accounted for some 2–16% of all deaths. Lung cancer occurs with all fibre types. There is no direct evidence that asbestos ingested in drinking water or food causes cancer, but the possibility remains.

Assessment of exposure

Environmental assessment

Exposure may be assessed by sampling static air at fixed locations by membrane filters, impingers, thermal precipitators, or konimeters. However, the most favoured method nowadays is personal air sampling by a membrane filter. Fibres of 5 μm or more in length (length/breadth ratio at least 3 : 1), collected from a membrane filter, should be counted by optical phase–contrast microscopy and expressed as number of fibres per ml of air sampled. In the case of other air samplers, total particles or fibres are expressed as number or mass of particles or fibres per unit volume of air. Quantification is also possible by X-ray diffraction or infrared spectrometry, the result being expressed in grams per volume of air sampled. Electron microscopy may be used to count fibres well below 0.1 μm diameter. This method is recommended for ambient air measurements when the fibres are virtually invisible under a light microscope. The levels of exposure of the general population are difficult to measure.

Biological assessment

Biochemical tests. A direct estimation of lung asbestos burden is only possible postmortem by first digesting and/or ashing the lung tissue and then counting or otherwise quantifying mineral fibres.

Radiography. Using the ILO *International Classification of Radiographs of Pneumoconioses*, pulmonary changes resulting from exposure to asbestos can be detected by radiography. The radiographic changes can be used to monitor exposure of the work force.

Respiratory function tests. These are useful, but are less specific than radiography.

Sputum test. Asbestos bodies in the sputum may be counted to give a rough estimate of relatively recent asbestos exposure.

Identification of fibre type

Optical X-ray or electron diffraction methods can distinguish chrysotile from amphiboles. To identify amphiboles, scanning or transmission electron microscopy coupled with energy-dispersive X-ray analysis is favoured.

Clinical effects

Asbestosis. Asbestosis is a chronic diffuse interstitial pulmonary fibrosis. Its severity is related to the length and intensity of exposure. In the early stages, the disease does not cause subjective symptoms. At physical examination, fine basal rales or crepitations may be found as an early sign. In advanced cases, the patient may suffer from dyspnoea and signs of respiratory insufficiency (cyanosis, clubbing of fingers, etc.) may develop. Radiographic signs are small irregular opacities with or without pleural thickening (variable).

Lung cancer. Asbestos-related lung cancer is clinically indistinguishable from lung cancer unrelated to asbestos exposure. Adenocarcinoma is reported to be more common in workers exposed to asbestos. Evidence of asbestosis is usually, but not invariably, present.

Malignant mesothelioma of the pleura. Chest pain and shortness of breath due to massive blood-stained pleural effusion frequently occur in pleural tumours. Peritoneal tumours generally give abdominal pain and swelling from gross ascites. In both cases the disease progresses rapidly to death, which occurs usually within a year of the first appearance of symptoms.

Other malignant diseases. Cancers of the gastrointestinal tract and possibly of the larynx may also occur, after prolonged exposure to asbestos. Clinically, these cancers are similar to gastrointestinal cancers of other etiology.

Exposure–effect relationships

Asbestosis

All evidence points to an increasing risk of asbestosis with exposure to rising concentrations of asbestos in air. The lack of agreed criteria for diagnosis makes it difficult to assess the exposure–response relationship. Clinical signs and symptoms, radiographic changes, reduction in pulmonary function, and deaths ascribed to asbestosis or to chronic respiratory disease have all been shown to be directly proportional to cumulative dust or fibre exposures, with little indication of a threshold. The disease usually develops after a long period of exposure to asbestos dust or fibre, seldom less than 5 years. In the past, poor working conditions in asbestos production, manufacture of asbestos products and other occupations involving exposure to asbestos fibres and dust have led to very high prevalence rates in workers employed for over 20 years.

Lung cancer

An exposure–response relationship, probably linear in nature, has been found in a number of epidemiological surveys. In mining and milling of chrysotile, over a working life of 40 years, the risk of lung cancer appears to rise by about 1.5% each time the air concentration of asbestos increases by 1 fibre/ml. In insulation work and manufacture of asbestos products, especially of textiles, the risk sometimes appears to be much higher (possibly tenfold or more) than that seen in mining and milling operations. Exposure to amphiboles probably carries a greater risk of cancer than does exposure to chrysotile. The cumulative risk of lung cancer in workers who smoke and who are exposed to asbestos is greater than the sum of the risks of lung cancer from smoking and from asbestos exposure separately.

Malignant mesothelioma of the pleura

There are few data on this subject. The risk is probably related to the dose. However, tumours have been seen to occur following occupational exposure to crocidolite of a duration as short as 6 weeks.

Other malignant diseases

Epidemiological findings suggest an increased incidence of gastrointestinal cancers following heavy exposure to asbestos, but exposure–response relationships are far from clear and other factors may be involved. Some, but not all, studies have suggested an association between asbestos exposure and laryngeal cancer, but there is no clear relationship between the incidence of the disease and the amount of exposure.

Prognosis

There is a gradual increase in symptoms and signs of pulmonary fibrosis even after the cessation of exposure. It has been shown that persons with pulmonary radiological changes are at an increased risk of death.

Differential diagnosis

Asbestosis in the absence of pleural thickening may be difficult to distinguish from chronic idiopathic diffuse interstitial pulmonary fibrosis. Minor radiographic parenchymal changes increase with age even in the absence of asbestos exposure.

Occupational history and specific radiographic changes in the lung are the only methods of determining whether a lung cancer seen in a worker is due to asbestos exposure. Pathologists often differ over the diagnosis of malignant mesothelioma of the pleura because it is difficult to distinguish this cancer from peripheral adenocarcinoma and metastatic pleural tumours.

Susceptibility

Variation in pulmonary response to asbestos exposure is suspected but has not yet been demonstrated. Studies of histocompatibility antigens (HL-A) have not identified any differences in susceptibility.

There is conflicting evidence on whether the risk of contracting asbestosis is affected by smoking. However, smokers apparently suffer greater disability and mortality. The risk of mesothelioma is unaffected by smoking.

Health examinations

Preplacement examination

The preplacement examination should include a medical history, a physical examination, chest X-ray, and lung function tests in order to establish baseline data for surveillance and to prevent persons with respiratory diseases from being exposed to asbestos.

Periodic examination

In medical terms the periodic examination is the same as the preplacement one. It should be carried out at intervals depending on the level of exposure at the workplace, age of the worker, and the results of previous health examinations.

Since it takes a long time for asbestosis to develop, 5-year intervals between health examinations may be appropriate during the first 10 years of work. Thereafter, the examinations should be more frequent.

The benefit to be derived from the early treatment of lung cancer is probably insufficient to warrant less than one-year intervals between routine X-rays. Because of the possibility of late development of asbestos-related diseases, supervision should continue even after the cessation of work involving exposure to asbestos.

Case management

If an asbestos-related disease is suspected, surveillance and control measures should be intensified, and workers should be fully informed of the risks and advised to avoid further exposure. Workers with signs of asbestosis should be informed about the disease, advised to stop smoking, and should be closely supervised. Advice concerning further employment entailing asbestos exposure depends on the age of the worker and individual circumstances.

Lung cancer should be treated as if unrelated to asbestos. There is no effective treatment for either asbestosis or malignant mesothelioma of the pleura.

Control measures

Regulations. Most industrialized countries have adopted an exposure limit of 2 fibres/ml of air (a few as little as 1 fibre/ml) as the maximum permissible time-weighted average concentration for chrysotile. The spraying of asbestos is now widely banned, and the use of crocidolite is also banned or severely restricted in some countries, with similar regulations for Amosite being under review. Some countries, however, make no distinction between different types of fibre. Concern remains that the hazard is not adequately reflected by fibre counts done with an optical microscope since by this method finer fibres, which are more dangerous, are not detected. As a result, the hazard may vary considerably in different industrial processes even when the optically assessed environmental concentration of asbestos is the same.

Engineering. Successful dust control begins with enclosing machines and applying local exhaust ventilation where openings are unavoidable. Other methods of dust control include: (*a*) isolation of "dirty" operations; (*b*) reduction in the number of employees exposed; and (*c*) changing manufacturing methods, (e.g., making asbestos yarn by wet suspension and extrusion). Substitution of asbestos by safer alternative materials should also be considered. Moreover, whenever possible, asbestos should be made wet before working with it. Also, asbestos could be treated with antidusting agents and asbestos yarn coated with polymer. Good housekeeping and the use of vacuum cleaners are essential. The use of respirators and protective clothing should be encouraged where it is impossible to avoid exposure. Shower and laundry facilities should be provided for workers in order to ensure that they leave the plant uncontaminated. All workers should be informed of the nature of the hazard and of methods of protection.

CHAPTER 3

Bronchopulmonary diseases caused by hard metal dusts

Properties of the causal agent

Hard metal is a term used for extremely hard sintered metal carbides of tungsten (to which small amounts of titanium, tantalum, vanadium, molybdenum, or chromium carbide have been added) bonded together by cobalt (also iron and nickel). The pulverized and compressed constituents are heated to a high temperature (1500 °C) and cooled abruptly.

Uses

Hard or sintered metals are used in the manufacture of tools, drills, and metal parts of particular hardness (90–95% that of diamond).

Occupations involving risk of exposure to hard metal dust

Workers at greatest risk are those engaged in the production of sintered carbides (mixing, pulverizing, forming, furnace heating, machining, precision grinding) and in the manufacture of tools and machine parts, as well as those responsible for sharpening the tools produced. Although those engaged in grinding and sharpening are the most exposed to the hazard, workers engaged in other tasks in the immediate vicinity in the same workshop may also run a high risk of exposure.

Mechanism of action

Absorption of hard metal dust takes place exclusively via the lungs. The absorbed dust is distributed to other parts of the body in the same way as other dust particles: insoluble dust particles are retained in the lung tissue, while the soluble components are carried by blood to other parts of the body. Only cobalt is excreted in small amounts in the urine.

26

Assessment of exposure

Environmental assessment

Both respirable and total dust concentrations should be measured, preferably by a personal sampler.

Biological assessment

Increased excretion of cobalt in the urine may be used as a supplementary test of environmental exposure. However, the relationship between hard metal dust exposure and cobalt in urine is obscure.

Clinical effects

In a majority of those exposed, a variety of irritative symptoms are seen, including cough, allergic rhinitis, asthma-like dyspnoea, and dyspnoea on exertion. The symptoms improve after the cessation of exposure. Diffuse interstitial pulmonary fibrosis is far less common and affects about 1–4 % of workers.

In general, the early signs of disease begin to appear following exposure for more than three years. These include dry cough, weight loss, progressive dyspnoea on exertion. Crepitant rales may be heard on auscultation. Chest X-rays, which are difficult to interpret at the onset of the disease, show linear markings and reticular shadows of varying opacity. Health examinations show classical symptoms of respiratory insufficiency, with a simultaneous decline in VC and $FEV_{1.0}$. Oxyhaemoglobin hyposaturation of the arterial blood occurs exclusively on exertion in the initial period and there is a decline in carbon monoxide diffusion.

Morphologically, there is alveolar and interstitial fibrosis, which produces an enlargement of the septa; thinned alveoli with cuboidal lining cells alternate with areas of emphysematous distension.

The part played by individual metals in the pathogenesis is still under discussion. Cobalt is the most toxic component under experimental conditions and is thought to play the dominant role. However, it is generally agreed that the association of tungsten with cobalt is responsible for the development of diffuse interstitial fibrosis.

Exposure–effect relationship

An airborne dust concentration of 100–6000 respirable particles per ml^3 of air has been found to cause the disease. Many metals are usually present in the dust: tungsten (67–90 %), cobalt (6–20 %), and tantalum, titanium, vanadium, iron, and niobium in amounts not exceeding 2 %.

Prognosis

Mostly there is a progressive aggravation, with respiratory insufficiency and right ventricular failure. However, in some patients the condition remains stable for several years (6–10 years), and some regression of the signs of the disease may be noted following withdrawal from exposure, at least at an early stage.

Differential diagnosis

Idiopathic diffuse interstitial fibrosis, Hamman–Rich syndrome, and fibrosis resulting from identified causes (including mineral dust pneumoconioses) should be excluded.

Susceptibility

Individuals with allergic and other respiratory diseases (especially asthma) may be considered as specially vulnerable.

Health examinations

Preplacement examination

The preplacement examination should include a medical history and a physical examination in order to identify persons with allergic skin and respiratory diseases. A chest X-ray should be taken and basic pulmonary function tests (FVC, $FEV_{1.0}$) should be carried out.

Periodic examination

In medical terms the periodic examination is the same as the preplacement one. This test should be repeated annually, and if any abnormality is found, appropriate lung-function tests should be done.

Screening test

Pulmonary function tests (FVC, $FEV_{1.0}$) should be done every six months.

Case management

On suspicion of disease, the individual should be temporarily withdrawn from exposure (till clarification). If the disease is confirmed he should be permanently excluded from work involving hard-metal dust exposure.

Control measures

The exposure of workers must be controlled by appropriate technical measures (enclosing machines and applying local exhaust ventilation, etc.) in order to reduce dust concentrations below the recommended exposure limits. The use of personal protective devices (respirators) may be necessary during work operations involving exposure to very high concentrations of dust.

The exposure limit adopted in most countries for soluble compounds of tungsten is 1 mg/m^3 of air and for insoluble compounds 5 mg/m^3 of air (as tungsten); for cobalt metal fumes and dust, the exposure limit is 0.1–0.5 mg/m^3 of air.

CHAPTER 4

Bronchopulmonary diseases caused by cotton dust, flax, hemp, or sisal dust: byssinosis

Properties of the causal agents

Byssinosis is caused by exposure to airborne dusts of cotton, flax, and soft hemp. Cotton dust is composed of four fractions: cellulose fibre; plant debris (tiny broken cotton leaves and bracts); earthy matter (soil); and saprophytic microorganisms (usually Gram-negative bacteria and fungi that grow on the cotton during storage). The relative proportion of each depends on the circumstances of cotton harvesting and storage. Hand-picked cotton has less plant debris than cotton harvested by machines and fresh cotton has fewer microorganisms than stored cotton.

Airborne dust in flax and soft hemp is usually composed of plant debris and microorganisms that grow on flax during retting.

Occurrence and uses

Cotton, flax, hemp, and sisal are grown in many parts of the world. Industrial processing of cotton involves various operations: (*a*) ginning, in which cotton seeds are separated from lint; (*b*) bale pressing (in exporting countries); and (*c*) cotton manufacturing, which involves bale opening, blowing, carding, spinning, preparation of yarn, and weaving. All these operations are usually dusty. Airborne dust from weaving differs from that produced in earlier processes and contains particles of the sizing material. Cotton waste is used to produce cotton wool, which is almost entirely composed of clean cellulose fibres. The remaining waste contains a high proportion of earthy matter and plant debris.

In the processing of flax, the first operation is the retting of the dried flax plant in water tanks. Then, the flax fibres are dried and broken in order to separate the fibres for spinning and weaving. The last three operations are usually dusty.

Occupations involving risk of byssinosis

Workers in the textile industry carrying out dusty operations are at greatest risk. In some developing countries, flax breaking and spinning are performed at home, causing dust exposure to the workers and their families.

Mechanism of action

The pathogenesis of byssinosis is not as yet fully clear. There is evidence that a toxic histamine-releasing substance may be responsible for the typical symptoms of byssinosis, namely respiratory tightness on the first day of work after the weekend holiday. It is widely believed that this histamine-releasing action of cotton dust is caused by a water-soluble, heat stable, small molecular compound derived from the bracts of the cotton plant.

In addition to histamine release, exposure to cotton dust causes irritation in the upper respiratory tracts and bronchi, which after prolonged exposure slowly progresses to chronic obstructive pulmonary disease.

It is also likely that there is more than one type of human reaction to these dusts. Endotoxins found in Gram-negative bacteria have been shown to cause byssinosis-like symptoms on inhalation.

Assessment of exposure

The best means of assessing exposure to cotton, flax, and hemp dust is by gravimetric evaluation of airborne dust, either as a whole or only the respirable fraction. Various size-selective samplers are currently in use. However, the best of these is the vertical elutriator sampler. Gravimetric personal dust samplers for sampling respirable dust of cotton and flax below 10 μm particle size are also available.

Clinical effects

In the early stages, byssinosis is characterized by symptoms of chest tightness (usually towards the end of the work-shift) on the first day of work after the weekend break or after holidays. There is often a decline in $FEV_{1.0}$, which may be symptomless in some workers. Within one or two days, most symptoms tend to disappear, except for irritation in the upper respiratory tract. As the disease progresses, the chest tightness is accompanied by breathlessness, the symptoms becoming worse and persisting for a longer time. In its late stages, the disease resembles chronic bronchitis and emphysema, except for the history of chest tightness and decline in ventilatory capacity, characteristically worse at the beginning of the work week. Chest X-rays do not show any specific changes, nor has any specific pathology been identified in the lungs of workers who have died from this disease.

Exposure–effect relationship

Prevalence rates of byssinosis varying from 20 % to 50 % have been reported in cotton cardrooms with respirable dust concentrations between 0.35 mg/m³ and 0.60 mg/m³. Prevalences of less than 10 % occur only in workrooms with respirable dust concentrations of less than 0.1 mg/m³. However, in one study in ginning workers (who usually work seasonally) chest tightness at the beginning of seasonal work was reported in 19 % of workers exposed to respirable dust concentrations of 0.11 mg/m³. Thus, even when concentrations of respirable dust are as low as about 0.1 mg/m³, symptoms may occur in a sizeable proportion of workers after return from an annual holiday.

Prognosis

The decline in ventilatory capacity during the work-shift is a temporary phenomenon, and in the early stages it is reversible. But follow-up studies show a greater decline of $FEV_{1.0}$ per year among textile workers with a long history of dust exposure than among unexposed subjects.

Differential diagnosis

There are three criteria for the clinical diagnosis of byssinosis: (a) history of proven exposure to cotton, flax, hemp, and sisal dust; (b) symptoms of byssinosis as identified by a standard questionnaire,[1] and in some cases, by the clinical manifestations of chronic bronchitis; and (c) drop in ventilatory capacity during the work-shift, which is greater in those suffering from byssinosis than in normal individuals and is generally higher on the first day of the working week than on other days.

Susceptibility

Smokers seem to be more susceptible to byssinosis than non-smokers. They are also more likely to suffer from advanced forms of the disease.

---

[1] See WHO Technical Report Series, No. 684, 1983.

Health examinations

Preplacement examination

The preplacement health examination should include a medical history and a physical examination, with special attention to atopy and allergic and respiratory diseases. Chest X-ray and basic pulmonary function test (VC, $FEV_{1.0}$) should also be carried out.

Periodic examination

In medical terms the periodic examination is the same as the preplacement one. It should be repeated usually once a year. A questionnaire for byssinosis should be included in the examination.

In groups of workers, a drop of more than 10 % in $FEV_{1.0}$ during the work-shift on the day after the weekend holiday may provide advance warning that workers are liable to develop byssinosis. Note that this applies only to groups of workers where the statistical significance of the decline in $FEV_{1.0}$ can be evaluated against controls.

Case management

The early cases of byssinosis should be moved to work involving less exposure. In these cases, the symptoms usually disappear. Advanced cases with obstructive pulmonary disease should be removed from dust exposure altogether and given appropriate therapy.

Control measures

These mainly involve dust suppression by enclosing dusty operations (gins) and providing appropriate ventilation (e.g., suction stripping equipment together with downwards exhaust ventilation).

There have been trials of washing and steaming the cotton before processing, but these have not proved to be very effective in eliminating the diseases.

Personal protective equipment such as filter masks is useful if it is checked regularly for effective and complete air filtration. Unfortunately, the wearing of masks is inconvenient, particularly in hot climates.

The exposure limits for total airborne dust vary in different countries from 2 mg/m³ to 6 mg/m³ of air. The recommended health-based occupational exposure limits (time-weighted averages) for inhalable dust, as measured by the vertical elutriator with a cut-off point of 15 μm, are: for cotton ginning 0.5 mg/m³; for cotton yarn processing, carding, spinning, etc. 0.2 mg/m³; and for cotton weaving

0.75 mg/m^3. For flax, a tentative value of 2 mg/m^3, and in workplaces with green or chemically-retted (not dew- or water-retted) flax, a value of 5 mg/m^3 have been recommended. For soft hemp, a tentative value of 2 mg/m^3 has been recommended.

CHAPTER 5

Occupational asthma

Properties of the causal agent

Occupational asthma is caused by the inhalation of sensitizing agents or irritants present in the working environment, such as dusts, droplets and gases. The list of causal agents is very long and only the major classes are mentioned here.

Sensitizing agents

These substances cause bronchial hyperreaction. They include: material of plant origin (e.g., grain, flour, coffee beans, castor beans, colophony (rosin), tea fluff, tobacco, woods such as red cedar, and mansonia); dusts from shellfish and laboratory animals (e.g., rats, mice, guinea-pigs) and from mites, silkworms, and other insects; metals (particularly their salts) such as platinum, chromium, and nickel; organic compounds (formaldehyde, phenylenediamine, isocyanates, particularly toluene diisocyanate, trimellitic anhydride, phthalic anhydride, epoxy resins, reactive dyes, and many others); and drugs (particularly antibiotics) and enzymes (detergents derived from *Bacillus subtilis*, pepsin, papain, etc.).

Irritants

Irritants cause chemical asthma. They include: strong alkalis, acids, oxidizing agents (ammonia, chlorine, hydrogen chloride, phosgene, hydrogen fluoride, oxides of nitrogen or sulfur, zinc chloride, etc.); and inert dust (non-fibrous and non-toxic dust) in extreme concentrations.

Occurrence and uses

The above-mentioned agents are used in many industrial processes, some of them appearing as undesirable admixtures. They are encountered mainly in: food production and processing; wood and furniture industry; animal breeding; engineering works; chemical industry; construction work (insulation, painting, etc.); fur processing (dyes); pharmaceutical industry; health facilities; and production of detergents.

35

Occupations involving risk of exposure

Workers at greatest risk include: those who handle grains and cereals (silo workers, millers, bakers); grain storage workers exposed to mites; workers exposed to dusts from castor or coffee beans and those involved in tea sifting and packing; woodworkers, sawmill operators, and workers in the furniture industry; printing workers; laboratory workers handling animals; manufacturers of detergent enzymes, platinum refiners, (rarely chromium or nickel platers); workers in the chemical and pharmaceutical industries; manufacturers of polyurethane foam using isocyanates; painters and insulation workers; meat wrappers exposed to fumes of polyvinyl chloride (PVC) soft-wrap film; and health personnel.

Mechanism of action

The respiratory disorders caused by sensitizing agents and irritants are characterized by: (*a*) acute reversible obstruction of the airways caused by bronchoconstriction, airway oedema or inflammation; and (*b*) mucous excretion induced by exposure to agents inherent in the work processes. Clinically, these disorders do not differ from other types of asthma. In some circumstances the same agents may cause allergic alveolitis.

Most of the sensitizing agents stimulate the production of a specific immunoglobulin (IgE) in susceptible individuals (type I hypersensitivity). In non-atopic subjects, hypersensitivity may be mediated by short-term sensitizing immunoglobulin antibody. Allergens that give rise to these responses include grain dust, animal products, insect proteins, enzymes derived from *B. subtilis*, gum acacia, and castor oil beans. They usually provoke an immediate asthmatic reaction, starting within a few minutes to 30 minutes after exposure. Delayed reaction may occur some four to eight hours after exposure, sometimes in combination with the immediate reaction. Although such an asthmatic reaction is usually indicative of type III hypersensitivity, it is uncertain to what extent this is a cause of asthma in occupational exposures.

Substances of small molecular mass (metallic ions, isocyanates) may act as haptens and form complete allergens, causing asthma-like symptoms. There is some evidence that non-immunological mechanisms may also play a role, e.g., by histamine release from the mast cells.

Irritants act by causing direct tissue injury. An asthma-like reaction may also be caused by exposure to heavy concentrations of inert dust, particularly in individuals with increased nonspecific bronchial reactivity.

Assessment of exposure

Environmental assessment

In the case of irritants, it is important to assess their concentrations in the air by the usual methods of environmental assessment. However, for agents causing hypersensitivity reactions this may not be necessary, because even minute amounts of allergens can give rise to acute symptoms.

Biological assessment

Reliable biological tests of exposure are available for only a limited number of chemical substances. If there is a relevant antigen, skin tests and IgE estimations may indicate hypersensitivity in symptom-free workers, reflecting the allergenic potency of the agent.

Clinical effects

The clinical symptoms of bronchial hyperreaction and chemical asthma are identical to those of asthma of non-occupational origin. They include: dyspnoea, chest tightness, wheezing, and pulmonary function impairment of the obstructive type. Chest X-rays show no signs of pathology. With an immediate hypersensitivity reaction, the attack develops within a few minutes after exposure at the workplace itself, and the patient recovers within about two hours after withdrawal from exposure. The late hypersensitivity reaction starts several hours after the first exposure, often after the work-shift or at night, and recovery may take more than 24 hours.

Asthmatic attacks caused by irritants usually develop during or immediately after the exposure. Some of the irritants may induce effects after a latency period of many hours (e.g., oxides of nitrogen).

Exposure–effect relationship

There is generally a good correlation between the concentration of irritants in the air and adverse effects. No such relationship exists for sensitizing agents.

Prognosis

Although in most individuals asthmatic symptoms cease if there is no further exposure, in some subjects prolonged asthma may ensue in the absence of further occupational contact with the causative agent. In such cases, continuing environmental contact with an ubiquitous agent, non-specific irritation, or cross-reactivity with other non-occupational allergens should be suspected.

If after the first attack of asthma the patient is not withdrawn from further exposure, progressive deterioration of asthmatic symptoms and of lung function may result.

Differential diagnosis

The first step is to differentiate bronchial asthma from other causes of transitory dyspnoea (respiratory, cardiovascular). The second task is to identify the (occupational) etiology of asthma (see also Part 3). In diagnosing asthma-like symptoms in workers the following points should be kept in mind:

—a great variety of occupational exposures are capable of inducing asthma;

—the possibility of an occupational origin of asthma should be considered in atopic persons when no extrinsic factor is readily identifiable; and

—the possibility of a late asthmatic reaction (several hours after exposure, at home or at night) should always be considered.

The diagnostic methods given below have proved useful.

—*Skin prick reaction with the suspected allergen.* It should be pointed out here that the correlation between a positive skin reaction and asthma is rather low.

—*Serological tests with specific IgE antibodies against certain substances* (e.g., *B. subtilis* enzymes, platinum, isocyanates).

—*Bronchial provocation tests.* Nonspecific tests of bronchial hyper-activity (e.g., inhalation of histamine or acetylcholine derivatives) are less reliable than inhalation tests with suspected allergen taken from the workplace. To detect delayed reactions, a clinical examination and lung function tests ($FEV_{1.0}$) should be carried out repeatedly during 24 hours after exposure.

—*Re-exposure of the worker at the workplace during a symptom-free period.* This test can confirm the diagnosis of occupational asthma without identifying the causal agent. A physical examination and lung function tests should be carried out before and after re-exposure.

Susceptibility

Atopic subjects and those with chronic inflammatory diseases of the respiratory tract are particularly susceptible.

Health examinations

Preplacement examination

The preplacement examination should include a medical history (with special attention to atopy of skin and the respiratory system), a physical examination, and simple lung function tests.

Periodic examinations

In medical terms the periodic examination is the same as the preplacement examination. It is usually carried out at one year intervals.

Case management

Individuals with identified occupational asthma should be removed from work involving exposure to the agent responsible. Desensitization is difficult to achieve.

Control measures

Technical measures should be applied to control the concentration of air pollutants in the working environment. Personal protective devices (respirators, etc.) may be necessary in some operations. Safe alternatives to irritants and sensitizing agents should be sought.

CHAPTER 6

Extrinsic allergic pneumonitis

Extrinsic allergic pneumonitis is a general term for a group of disorders caused by a hypersensitivity reaction to inhaled dust, especially dust containing material of fungal origin.

Properties of the causal agent

Dust containing organic antigens (particularly thermophilic micro-organisms and moulds) or animal proteins is the main cause of this disease. The same agents may also cause bronchial hyperreaction (see Chapter 5).

The most common types of dust, responsible antigens, and the resulting clinical conditions are summarized in Table 1.

Occupations involving risk of extrinsic allergic pneumonitis

Workers in agriculture, beverage industries (breweries), wood and furniture industries, and animal keepers are at greatest risk.

Mechanism of action

Inhaled dust particles that are small enough to be retained in the alveoli and small airways and that contain antigenic material are responsible for the disease. In the early acute phase, the walls of the alveoli and small airways are infiltrated with lymphocytes and there is characteristic formation of sarcoid-type granulomata. The chronic phase is characterized by diffuse interstitial pulmonary fibrosis.

Assessment of exposure

Environmental assessment

The usual methods for the determination of concentrations of pollutants in air as well as microbiological methods for the identification of microorganisms are used.

Table 1. Causal agents of extrinsic allergic pneumonitis[a]

Type of dust	Responsible antigen	Disease
Mouldy hay	*Micropolyspora faeni* *Thermoactinomyces vulgaris*	Allergic pneumonitis due to *Micropolyspora faeni* Allergic pneumonitis due to *Thermoactinomyces vulgaris*
Mouldy bagasse	*Thermoactinomyces vulgaris*	Bagasse pneumonitis
Mushroom compost	*Micropolyspora faeni* *Thermoactinomyces vulgaris*	Allergic pneumonitis due to *Micropolyspora faeni* Allergic pneumonitis due to *Thermoactinomyces vulgaris*
Cork dust	Cork dust	Allergic pneumonitis due to cork dust
Maple bark	*Cryptostroma corticale*	Maple-bark allergic pneumonitis
Redwood sawdust	*Graphium* *Pullaria*	Allergic pneumonitis due to graphium
Wood pulp	*Alternaria*	Allergic pneumonitis due to wood dust
Mouldy barley	*Aspergillus clavatus* *Aspergillus fumigatus*	Allergic aspergillosis
Mouldy straw	*Aspergillus versicolor*	Allergic aspergillosis
Pigeon, parrot, and other bird droppings	Sera, protein and droppings	Avian-antigen allergic pneumonitis
Wheat flour	*Sitophilus granarius*	Allergic pneumonitis due to *Sitophilus granarius*
Animal hairs		Animal-hair allergic pneumonitis
Coffee bean	Coffee bean dust	Allergic pneumonitis due to coffee bean dust
Paprika		Allergic pneumonitis due to paprika dust

[a] Adapted from: KEY, M. M. ET AL. *Occupational diseases.* Washington, DC, US Department of Health, Education, and Welfare, 1977.

Biological assessment

The presence of specific precipitins in the sera of symptom-free workers may indicate past exposure and the risk of disease.

Clinical effects

Acute and subacute disease

Symptoms develop about 4–8 hours after heavy exposure to dust containing the antigen. They include: headache, fever, nausea, vomiting, chest tightness, breathlessness, and cough. There may be cyanosis and crepitations on auscultation. In advanced cases, chest X-rays show small opacities distributed throughout the middle and lower areas of the lungs. The diminution of ventilatory capacity and gas transfer are the main lung function impairments.

Chronic disease

After repeated acute episodes, and rarely without an antecedent acute episode, recurrent exposures to low concentrations of antigenic dust gradually lead to dyspnoea. Lung function tests reveal restrictive ventilatory defect and impaired gas transfer. Chest X-rays show a variety of dispersed linear opacities corresponding to the development of diffuse interstitial pulmonary fibrosis.

Exposure–effect relationships

The exposure–effect relationship between allergic dust exposure and extrinsic allergic pneumonitis has not yet been established.

Prognosis

Acute disease is usually reversible within several weeks. However, it may progress into the chronic form, particularly if the exposure does not cease. Chronic disease may steadily worsen and result in congestive heart failure.

Differential diagnosis

Acute disease should be distinguished from acute respiratory infections (viral, bacterial) and pneumonitis due to nitrogen dioxide (silo-fillers' disease). In the chronic phase, other causes of diffuse interstitial pulmonary fibrosis should be excluded, e.g., tuberculosis, sarcoidosis, pneumoconioses due to mineral dust, and Hamman-Rich syndrome. Lung biopsy may be necessary. Specific precipitins are present in most acute cases; a smaller proportion of chronic cases also show specific precipitins.

Susceptibility

Only a small proportion of workers exposed to dust containing antigens develop extrinsic allergic pneumonitis. The reasons for susceptibility have not yet been identified. The level of exposure may play a role.

Health examinations

Preplacement examination

A preplacement medical examination is of limited value in the occupational groups at risk.

Periodic examinations

This is also of limited value in the occupational groups at risk.

Case management

Immediate removal from exposure should be the first step. Treatment with corticosteroids is valuable, particularly when the pneumonitis is acute.

Control measures

Changes should be made in work practices in order to avoid the multiplication of moulds and bacteria. Technical measures should be applied to control dust in the air of workplaces. Personal protective devices (respirators, etc.) may be necessary in particularly dusty operations.

CHAPTER 7

Diseases caused by beryllium and its toxic compounds

Properties of the causal agent

Beryllium is a light grey metal slightly soluble in dilute acids and alkalis.

Occurrence and uses

Beryllium for industrial use is obtained from the mineral beryl. Beryllium and its alloys are widely used in the aerospace industry and in the manufacture of precision instruments and computers, non-arcing cutters for the petroleum industry, X-ray tubes, fluorescent tubes, vacuum electrodes, heater cathodes, and moderators for use in nuclear reactors.

Occupations involving exposure to beryllium and its toxic compounds

Beryllium alloy workers, cathode-ray-tube makers, aircraft and spacecraft technicians, and nuclear reactor workers are at greatest risk of exposure.

Mechanism of action

Absorption

The main route of entry into the body is via the respiratory tract. There is some absorption from the gastrointestinal tract and through undamaged skin, but it is of no practical importance.

Distribution

Most of the beryllium and its insoluble compounds that enter the body are fixed in the lungs. Soluble compounds are gradually redistributed to other organs. Beryllium may cross the placenta and reach the fetus; it may also be passed to infants in the breast milk of nursing mothers.

Excretion

Beryllium is eliminated via urine and faeces.

Assessment of exposure

Environmental assessment

Both respirable and total dust concentrations should be measured, preferably with a personal sampler.

Biological assessment

Beryllium is sometimes present in the urine of persons not occupationally exposed in concentrations of usually less than 1 mg/litre. In groups of exposed workers the concentrations are higher, but they do not necessarily correlate with the amount of exposure or severity of lung disease. In the absence of clinical signs and symptoms, the presence of beryllium in biological materials is not a sign of disease. At autopsy, beryllium may be found in the organs of persons long after the cessation of exposure. However, there is little correlation between the amount of beryllium found in the lungs and the presence of disease.

Clinical effects

Soluble beryllium compounds (chloride, sulfate, fluoride) may cause acute intoxication, while relatively insoluble forms (metallic beryllium and beryllium oxide) cause chronic disease.

Acute berylliosis arises from accidental inhalation of high amounts of soluble beryllium compounds. It manifests itself as nasopharyngitis, tracheobronchitis, bronchiolitis, or pulmonary oedema, appearing from a few hours to 1–2 days after exposure.

Chronic berylliosis is caused by slightly soluble beryllium compounds. The allergenic effect of beryllium has a major role in the pathogenesis of berylliosis: it causes the disease by inducing an immunopathological process in susceptible individuals. The disease may develop many years after the cessation of beryllium exposure. A distinctive granulomatous process, which is mainly confined to the lungs, but which may also be found in other organs (liver, spleen, etc.), is typical. The usual early signs and symptoms are breathlessness on exertion, cough, and fever; later on there may be asthenia and rapid weight loss.

The disease may progress rapidly under certain conditions (e.g., surgery, respiratory infection, or pregnancy). Respiratory or cardiac insufficiency may develop. Lung X-rays show diffuse bilateral granulomatosis or, in early stages, only enlarged lymph nodes. The respiratory function is impaired largely by reduction in the diffusion capacity of the lungs, which is detectable in early stages of the disease.

Delayed effects

In animal experiments, beryllium is a carcinogen. Scarcity of data led the International Agency for Research on Cancer to include beryllium and its compounds in the group of probable carcinogens for man.

Exposure–effect relationship

Although berylliosis usually results from high exposure to beryllium and its compounds, sometimes even a brief contact with low concentrations is sufficient to bring on the disease; it may even develop after the cessation of exposure. Thus, there is no systematic exposure–effect relationship.

Prognosis

In acute berylliosis recovery usually takes 2–6 weeks. However, sometimes there may be permanent damage (bronchitis, sytemic sclerosis involving the lung). Chronic berylliosis may be symptom-free or rapidly progressive and severely disabling.

Differential diagnosis

Sarcoidosis, other pneumoconioses, Hamman-Rich syndrome, miliary tuberculosis, and miliary carcinomatosis should be excluded. Lung biopsy may be necessary. While some specialists consider allergy tests on skin with a solution of beryllium salts as sensitive diagnostic methods, others fear such tests may cause undue sensitization of the subject. Diagnosis must be supported by a history of exposure.

Susceptibility

Atopic subjects and persons with respiratory diseases are considered by some as specially vulnerable.

Health examinations

Preplacement examination

The preplacement health examination should include a medical history and a physical examination, with special attention to atopy and allergic skin respiratory diseases. Chest X-ray and basic pulmonary function tests (VC, $FEV_{1.0}$) are also essential.

Periodic examination

In medical terms the periodic examination is the same as the preplacement one.

Case management

In acute berylliosis, contact with beryllium must be discontinued immediately. Since mild symptoms may precede a severe attack, the patient should be admitted to hospital. Chelating agents to eliminate beryllium have been tried. Pulmonary oedema, cardiovascular insufficiency, and lung infections must be prevented.

Corticosteroids may have a beneficial effect in chronic berylliosis but they must be continued indefinitely. Any further contact with beryllium must cease.

Control measures

The exposure of workers to beryllium must be restricted by appropriate technical control measures as well as by personal protection measures including: wearing a respirator in areas with high beryllium content; working in a pressurized suit in particularly hazardous places; compulsory changing of working clothing; and wearing goggles, gloves, etc.

Exposure limits for beryllium in air in different countries range from 1 μg/m³ to 2 μg/m³.

CHAPTER 8

Diseases caused by cadmium and its toxic compounds

Properties of the causal agent

Cadmium is a soft, ductile, white metal with a bluish tinge. Its relatively low boiling point of 767 °C permits it to burn easily to form cadmium oxide fumes.

Occurrence and uses

Cadmium is mainly recovered from zinc, lead–zinc, and lead–copper–zinc ore. It is mainly used for electroplating of other metals. Large amounts of cadmium and its compounds are used as pigments and stabilizers in plastics. Cadmium is also used in nickel–cadmium batteries, low-melting alloys, and silver solders.

Occupations involving risk of cadmium exposure

Workers in primary or secondary cadmium smelters, cadmium plating industries, and alkaline battery factories, as well as cadmium pigment makers and users and welders are at greatest risk.

Since cadmium is a naturally occurring element and since some of its applications cause its wide dispersal in the environment, every human being is exposed to cadmium in food, air, and water. Cadmium exposure may also occur through tobacco smoking, chewing, etc.

Mechanism of action

Absorption

Cadmium may enter the body via the pulmonary or the oral route. The deposition rate in lungs (alveolar bed) varies inversely with particle size (approximately 50% of inhaled particles have a mean mass diameter of 0.1 μm and 20% of particles 2 μm). Thus, deposition is maximum when freshly generated cadmium fumes are inhaled. About 60% of cadmium deposited in the lower respiratory tract as cadmium oxide may be absorbed; absorption is probably less in the case of cadmium compounds of low solubility, such as cadmium sulfide.

The average oral absorption rate of cadmium has been estimated at 5%.

Distribution

Cadmium is efficiently retained in the body, bound mainly to metallothionein, a metal-binding protein of low molecular weight. It accumulates mainly in the liver and kidneys.

Excretion

Cadmium is mainly excreted via the urine and, to a lesser extent, by other routes (bile, gastrointestinal tract, saliva, hair, nails).

Assessment of exposure

Environmental assessment

Both respirable and total dust concentrations should be measured, preferably by a personal sampler. Since cadmium may be ingested and absorbed in the gastrointestinal tract, its concentration in air may not necessarily reflect the amount absorbed.

Biological assessment

In the absence of kidney damage, the cadmium level in urine reflects mainly the body burden of cadmium. Cadmium concentration in blood mainly indicates the exposure to cadmium during the last few months before blood sampling. In adults not exposed occupationally to the metal, it is extremely rare to find concentrations exceeding 0.5 μg cadmium per 100 ml of whole blood and 2 μg of cadmium per litre of urine (corrected for the specific gravity of urine of 1016 or a creatinine concentration of 1 g/litre).

Clinical effects

Acute poisoning

The principal acute manifestations following high-level exposure are gastrointestinal disturbances (after ingestion) and chemical asthma (after inhalation of cadmium oxide fumes).

Chronic poisoning

Various body organs may be affected after long-term exposure to cadmium. The critical organ (the site of earliest functional disturbance) is the kidney. Classically, the functional disturbances involve the proximal tubule, giving rise to a tubular type proteinuria (excretion of low molecular mass proteins such as β_2-microglobulin and retinol-binding protein) while the total proteinuria may still be within the normal range. In some workers, increased excretion of high-molecular-mass proteins (probably resulting from glomerular dysfunction) may accompany or even precede the excretion of low-molecular-mass proteins. Proteinuria may be associated with glycosuria, aminoaciduria, impaired acid excretion, decreased urine-concentrating capacity of the kidney, increased excretion of calcium and phosphorus, and increased plasma creatinine. Calciuria may lead to the development of renal stones.

Various types of lung disturbance (emphysema, obstructive pulmonary disease, diffuse interstitial fibrosis) have been reported in workers chronically exposed to cadmium dust and cadmium oxide fumes. Bone lesions (osteomalacia, osteoporosis, spontaneous fracture) constitute rare late manifestations of severe chronic intoxication. Other signs and symptoms have been attributed to cadmium exposure in industry, mainly anosmia, ulceration of the nasal mucosa, yellow coloration of the dental neck, mild anaemia, and slight liver dysfunction.

Delayed effects

Some epidemiological studies have suggested increased incidence of prostate cancer and possibly also of lung cancer, but the risk, if any, is low and probably reflects very high exposure in the past. The role of cadmium in the development of hypertension is still controversial.

Exposure–effect relationship

According to a WHO Study Group, exposure of less than 1 hour to cadmium oxide fumes and dust at a concentration not exceeding 250 µg Cd/m^3 of air would not lead to the occurrence of any lung reaction in workers with normal lung function.[1] To prevent any pulmonary effect of cadmium in long-term occupational exposure, the time-weighted average airborne concentration of cadmium oxide fumes or respirable dust should not exceed 20 µg Cd/m^3 (for a weekly exposure of 40 hours during the whole working life). To prevent renal dysfunction, the amount of cadmium in the renal cortex should be kept below 200 mg/kg wet weight. This corresponds to urinary excretion rate of 10 µg Cd/g of creatinine. For blood, a value of 10 µg Cd/litre of whole blood is proposed as a no-adverse-effect level for long-term exposure.

---

[1] WHO Technical Report Series, No. 647, 1980, p. 33.

Prognosis

Cadmium-related proteinuria and renal dysfunction are usually of slow progression and may result in renal failure. It is not yet established whether early proteinuria is reversible after the cessation of exposure.

Differential diagnosis

The presence of other renal diseases should be excluded. The typical biochemical pattern of cadmium-related proteinuria and the evidence of high cadmium body burden should be decisive factors in the diagnosis of cadmium poisoning.

Susceptibility

Persons showing lung disturbances (obstructive pulmonary disease, chronic bronchitis, emphysema, etc.), kidney damage, cardiovascular disease, and significantly increased cadmium body burden (possibly due to occupational exposure) are more susceptible than others.

Health examinations

Preplacement examination

The preplacement examination should include a medical history and a physical examination, with special attention to renal and respiratory systems and to exposure to health hazards such as tobacco, silica, asbestos, cotton dust, irritant gases, mercury, and lead. Analysis of urine for proteinuria and glycosuria and a microscopic examination of the sediment should also be done, along with a chest X-ray. Lung function tests should be performed (at least FVC and $FEV_{1.0}$ should be determined). If indicated, the tests recommended for periodic examinations (see below) should be done.

Periodic examinations

With the exception of chest X-ray, the entire preplacement examination should be repeated every 1–3 years. Additional tests include: (a) prostate palpation in men over 40; (b) cadmium concentration in urine and blood; (c) quantitative determination of total protein (biuret method), albumin, retinol-binding protein, and β_2-microglobulin concentrations in urine (see also Chapter 34, p. 231). (d) pulmonary symptomatology, assessed preferably by a standardized questionnaire; and (e) lung function tests (FVC and $FEV_{1.0}$).

Screening tests

The kidney function tests recommended for periodic examinations and FVC and $FEV_{1.0}$ should be done twice a year.

Case management

If the cadmium level in urine is found repeatedly to exceed 10–15 µg/g of urinary creatinine, the individual should be considered at risk of developing functional renal changes (not to be confounded with renal insufficiency). When increased excretion of protein in urine is found, a more extensive investigation of kidney function is recommended. Workers presenting any persistent signs of renal dysfunction should be removed from cadmium exposure. There is no specific treatment. Lung function disorders unexplained by age or smoking habit justify the removal of workers from cadmium exposure.

Control measures

Cadmium dust and fumes should be controlled by technical control measures. In order to prevent excessive inhalation of cadmium, particularly freshly generated cadmium fumes, respiratory protective devices may also be necessary when technical control measures alone are not adequate.

Workers should be informed of the risks associated with acute and long-term exposure to cadmium. A regular review of the appropriate control procedures is essential. Good personal hygiene practice for limiting undue ingestion of cadmium should be encouraged. These include, for example: change of clothes and showering before leaving the factory; removal of overalls before entering the factory canteen; wearing of gloves at work; not eating, drinking, smoking, or carrying cigarettes or pipes in work areas, and hand washing after work.

The exposure limits for cadmium in air in different countries vary from 0.01 mg/m³ to 0.05 mg/m³.

CHAPTER 9

Diseases caused by phosphorus and its toxic compounds

ELEMENTAL PHOSPHORUS AND ITS INORGANIC TOXIC COMPOUNDS

Properties of the causal agents

White (or yellow) phosphorus is a wax-like volatile solid that ignites spontaneously on coming into contact with air. Red phosphorus is a non-toxic solid allotrope of phosphorus. It is often contaminated by yellow phosphorus, and is of no industrial importance.

Phosphoric acid (H_3PO_4) may be solid or liquid. Phosphorus trichloride (PCl_3) and phosphorus pentachloride (PCl_5) occur as yellow fuming crystals. Phosphorus oxychloride ($POCl_3$) is a fuming liquid. Phosphorus pentasulfide (P_2S_5) is a crystalline solid. And phosphine (PH_3) is a gas with a garlic-like odour.

Occurrence and uses

Phosphorus occurs naturally in phosphate rocks. Yellow phosphorus is used for manufacturing red phosphorus, phosphorus alloys and compounds (such as phosphoric acid), metallic phosphides, munitions and pyrotechnics, and rodenticides. Extremely pure phosphorus is used in electronics for the manufacture of semiconductors. Phosphoric acid is used in the manufacture of phosphates (superphosphate fertilizers), pharmaceuticals, and in treating metals against rust. Phosphorus trichloride, phosphorus pentachloride, and phosphorus oxychloride are used as chlorinating agents in chemistry and in the production of other phosphates. Phosphorus pentachloride is also used as a catalyst in the production of acetylcellulose. Phosphorus pentasulfide is used in the manufacture of safety matches, ignition compounds, and organic syntheses of certain compounds. Phosphine is used as a fumigant insecticide and in the preparation of halides of phosphorus.

Occupations involving risk of exposure to phosphorus and its compounds

Bronze alloy makers, workers in the chemical industry (organic syntheses, fertilizers, pesticides, etc.), and fumigators are at greatest risk of exposure.

Mechanism of action

Absorption

In occupational exposure, absorption of phosphorus is almost exclusively by inhalation (gas, vapour, mist).

Biotransformation

Phosphorus and its compounds are metabolized in the body, mainly into phosphates.

Elimination

Volatile compounds of phosphorus are excreted to a minor extent in the exhaled air; the major part, however, is eliminated in the form of phosphates in urine.

Assessment of exposure

Environmental assessment

Air concentrations of phosphorus should be measured, preferably by means of personal sampling.

Biological assessment

No methods of biological assessment are available.

Clinical effects

Acute effects

Local effects. Skin contact with phosphorus may result in severe chemical burns. Phosphorus compounds are strong irritants to the skin, eyes, and the respiratory tract (feeling of burning, cough). Exposure to high concentrations of phosphorus may cause bronchitis or even pulmonary oedema.

Systemic effects. Acute poisoning usually occurs only when phosphorus is ingested accidentally or with suicidal intent. The initial shock is followed by damage to the liver, kidneys, heart muscle or small vessels. Systemic effects of phosphorus pentasulfide are similar to those of hydrogen sulfide (see Chapter 22). Phosphine causes dizziness, nausea, vomiting, headache, dyspnoea, and in severe cases, coma.

Chronic effects

Chronic phosphorus poisoning results from continuous absorption of small amounts of yellow phosphorus for several years; however, exposures shorter than one year have been reported in typical cases of chronic poisoning. Phosphorus mainly affects the skeletal system and liver. In the oral cavity, periostitis with suppuration and ulceration may develop, followed by bone necrosis and severe deformity of the mandible (phossy jaw), and less often the maxilla. Sequestration of bones may occur. Liver damage leads to toxic hepatitis, which is accompanied by dyspepsia, abdominal pain, cachexia, and jaundice.

Phosphorus compounds may cause chronic irritative or allergic dermatitis (see page 60), chronic nonspecific respiratory disease (dyspnoea, cough, phlegm, impairment of lung function), and conjunctivitis.

Exposure–effect relationship

No clear quantitative data are available. About 0.5 mg/m³ of phosphoric acid is irritant to unacclimatized subjects. The odour threshold of phosphine is about 0.3 mg/m³ which does not provide sufficient warning of dangerous concentrations.

Prognosis

The prognosis of local acute irritant effects depends on the severity of exposure and clinical signs. Pulmonary oedema may be fatal. The same is true of acute phosphorus poisoning resulting from ingestion of phosphorus. The prognosis of phossy jaw is unfavourable, and severe deformities may result. Toxic hepatitis may lead to lethal liver atrophy.

Differential diagnosis

Irritant effects on the respiratory tract should be differentiated from acute viral or bacterial bronchitis or bronchopneumonia and from lung oedema due to cardiac insufficiency. Work history and evidence of high-level exposure to phosphorus compounds are the most important factors in the diagnosis of phosphorus poisoning. Phossy jaw should be differentiated from other causes of periostitis or osteomyelitis. Toxic hepatitis should be distinguished from other liver damage (viral hepatitis, cirrhosis, etc.).

Susceptibility

Persons with chronic respiratory diseases, dermatitis, liver diseases, carious teeth, and poor dental hygiene are most susceptible.

Health examinations

Preplacement examination

The preplacement examination should include a medical history and a physical examination, with special attention to the eyes, respiratory system, teeth and gums, skeletal system, and liver (including basic biochemical tests described on page 229).

Periodic examination

In medical terms the periodic examination is the same as the preplacement one. In exposure to yellow phosphorus, the intervals between periodic examinations should not exceed 6 months. In exposure to phosphorus compounds, the interval is usually one year.

Case management

In acute poisoning, immediately remove the worker from exposure. If the eyes are affected, flush them with water, and if skin is contaminated, wash with soap and water. For skin and eye contact with phosphorus, a first aid procedure must be developed beforehand.

In order to prevent spontaneous combustion of phosphorus and local damage, washing of affected areas with a 20–50 g/litre copper sulfate solution, which coats the phosphorus with metallic copper, has been used. However, since this procedure involves the risk of copper absorption through the skin, washing of skin with a 20 g/litre silver nitrate solution has been recommended recently.

Respiratory irritation may need anti-inflammatory, antioedematous, broncholytic and anti-infection treatment. It may be necessary to observe the patient for 48–72 hours in order not to miss any delayed reactions. Necrosis of the mandible may require surgical treatment. Toxic hepatitis should be treated by the usual methods. Patients with chronic phosphorus poisoning should avoid any further work with phosphorus or with other hepatotoxic substances.

Control measures

Exposure should be reduced by technical control measures. Personal protective devices (gloves, aprons, shields, respirators, etc.) should be used whenever necessary.

The ranges of exposure limits in different countries for the concentrations of phosphorus and its compounds in workroom air are as follows: phosphorus (yellow) 0.03–0.1 mg/m^3; phosphoric acid 0.5–1 mg/m^3; phosphorus oxychloride 0.05–3 mg/m^3; phosphorus trichloride and pentachloride 0.2–1 mg/m^3; phosphorus pentasulfide 0.5–6 mg/m^3; and phosphine 0.1–0.4 mg/m^3.

ORGANOPHOSPHORUS COMPOUNDS

Properties of the causal agents

A large number of organophosphorus compounds has been synthetized for use as pesticides. Although their chemical structures vary considerably, they have a common physiological mechanism of action—inhibition of the enzyme cholinesterase. Organophosphorus pesticides are either esters of phosphoric, thiophosphoric, and dithiophosphoric acids or amides of pyrophosphoric, alkylphosphoric, alkylphosphonic, and fluorophosphoric acids. These compounds are solid crystalline or lucid, yellow-brown liquids, often of oily consistency. Many of them have a specific unpleasant odour. They are mostly heavier than water. Many are soluble in both organic solvents (oils, fats) and water. They are easily hydrolysed, particularly in alkaline media and at raised temperatures. Many are highly volatile.

Production and uses

Organophosphorus pesticides are produced and formulated (i.e., prepared in the form in which they are distributed to consumers) by the chemical industry. They are applied in fields, plantations, orchards, vineyards, forests, greenhouses, etc. to protect plants against pests (insects, sometimes rodents).

Occupations involving exposure to organophosphorus compounds

Laboratory and other workers involved in the synthesis or formulation of organophosphorus pesticides, spraymen, farm workers, and those responsible for stocking, transporting and distributing organophosphorus pesticides are at greatest risk of exposure.

Mechanism of action

Absorption

Organophosphorus compounds are absorbed into the body both by inhalation (vapours, aerosols) and by direct contact with skin.

Biotransformation

These compounds are highly soluble in biological media and easily pass across biological membranes and the blood–brain barrier. They undergo rapid biotransformation, particularly oxidation or enzymatic hydrolysis, followed by conjugation with glutathione. The intermediate metabolites may be less toxic (detoxication) or more toxic (activation) than the original substance.

The active compounds react with the enzyme cholinesterase. During this process, the molecule splits and the phosphorus-containing parts binds to cholinesterase (phosphorylation), rendering it inactive.

Excretion

The metabolites are excreted mainly in the urine.

Assessment of exposure

Environmental assessment

Methods for the determination of organophosphorus compounds in the air of workplaces (spectrophotometric, gas chromatographic) are available, but these can be used only in production or formulating plants (confined spaces). Personal sampling is preferable.

In field conditions, air sampling cannot be used to assess the concentration level precisely enough because of continuously changing conditions. In view of the possible skin absorption, skin-pad tests are useful in many work settings.

Biological assessment

There are two main methods: (*a*) determination of the activity of cholinesterase in blood, and (*b*) determination of the organophosphorus compound or its metabolites in biological material (urine, blood).

The most practical method of assessing exposure to organophosphorus insecticides is the determination of cholinesterase activity in blood. It is universal for all organophosphorus pesticides and reflects not only the level of exposure but also the intensity of biological effects. For screening purposes, several simple methods of measuring whole-blood and serum cholinesterase activity are used, and commercially produced tintometric kits or indicator paper tests are available. Since the above screening tests lack precision, methods based on spectrophotometric or pH-metric principles should be used whenever a more accurate assessment of exposure is required. With regard to these tests it should be noted that individual variations in cholinesterase activity reach $\pm 50\%$ from the average group value. It is therefore necessary to know the pre-exposure value of all individuals examined periodically.

There are two types of cholinesterase in blood: erythrocytic acetylcholinesterase or true cholinesterase (which is identical to that found in nervous tissues) and plasmatic cholinesterase (also called pseudocholinesterase). Both are inhibited by organophosphorus pesticides, but to different degrees, depending on the chemical properties of the pesticide. After poisoning, the plasmatic cholinesterase reactivates about two or three times faster than the erythrocytic cholinesterase. In periodic examinations, it is usual to determine the total blood cholinesterase activity. If inhibition is found, both erythrocytic and plasmatic enzyme activities should be determined separately. In the case of parathion poisoning, about 70% of the absorbed parathion is excreted in the urine as its metabolite, p-nitrophenol, whereas, in the case of fenitrothion, about 50–70% is excreted in the urine as p-nitro-m-cresol. The determination of these substances may be used as an exposure test. Many organophosphorus compounds or their metabolites can be determined in blood (by gas chromatography), but quantitative exposure tests based on this method have not yet been developed.

Biological effects

The main biological effect is the inhibition of various enzymes of the esterase group, particularly cholinesterases. This results in the accumulation of acetylcholine which in turn leads to the impairment of the transmission of nervous stimuli through nerve cells and ganglionic synapses. The basic symptomatology is usually divided into three groups: (a) stimulation of the parasympathetic nervous system—miosis, salivation, vomiting, diarrhoea, bronchial hypersecretion, and spasm; (b) muscular stimulation ranging from fasciculations to localized or generalized cramps; and (c) a varying degree of impairment of psychic functions and consciousness.

Some observations point to adverse effects on the fetus.

Clinical effects

Acute effects

After exposure to an organophosphorus compound, the onset of symptoms is usually prompt; sometimes, however, there may be a delay of up to 12 hours.

The sequence of the development of systemic effects varies with the route of entry of the compound. After exposure through inhalation, respiratory and ocular effects are the first to appear. Initial symptoms are headache, vertigo, blurring of vision, lacrimation, tightness in the chest, and salivation. There is miosis and heavy perspiration and auscultation of the lungs reveals wheezing and rales.

Gastrointestinal symptoms (nausea, abdominal pain, diarrhoea) are more common if the compound enters the body via the oral route. General symptoms include unrest, feeling of weakness in the limbs, and behavioural changes. Muscular fasciculations can be best seen on the eyelids, tongue, or muscles close to the site of skin absorption of the pesticide. Blood cholinesterase activity is inhibited to values of less than 40–50% of the pre-exposure level.

With severe intoxication, all symptoms and signs become aggravated. There is heavy dyspnoea, fasciculation, giddiness, confusion, and ataxia. In coma, there is loss of reflexes, Cheyne-Stokes respiration, convulsions, and eventually paralysis.

Chronic effects

The effects of chronic poisoning by organophosphorus pesticides are less well established. Some authorities claim that chronic exposure is characterized by persistent headache, vertigo, decreased memory, disturbance of sleep, loss of appetite, nausea, general weakness, and miosis. In severe cases, there is a decline in intellectual capacity and there may be short-term periods of disorientation of petit mal type and disseminated neurological signs.

In workers exposed to thiophos, cases of toxic hepatitis have been reported as well as slight increase in the number of neutrophilic leukocytes and toxic granulation of leukocytes. After exposure to metaphos and methylnitrophos, increased methaemoglobin level and slight anaemia with changes in the cardiovascular system have also been reported. The activity of cholinesterase is either unchanged or only slightly decreased. Some pesticides may induce chronic conjunctivitis or dermatitis of both the irritative and the allergic type. Also, other allergic phenomena such as bronchial asthma are possible.

Exposure–effect relationship

Clinical symptoms develop in sensitive subjects after their pre-exposure cholinesterase activity has dropped by 50–60%. The development of symptoms depends not only on the degree of cholinesterase inhibition, but also on the rate of inhibition. Mild, but rapid decrease in cholinesterase activity is often accompanied by clear clinical symptoms, whereas slow continuous decrease to the same values of activity may not cause any symptoms. Severe intoxication is always characterized by severe inhibition of cholinesterase activity, below 20% of the pre-exposure value, particularly in the activity of the plasmatic cholinesterase. There is some controversy regarding the development of the symptoms of chronic poisoning after exposure to atmospheric concentrations of organophosphorus compounds that do not themselves cause the inhibition of blood cholinesterase.

Prognosis

Although most of the mild cases of acute poisoning recover spontaneously in several days, lethal outcomes of severe poisonings are possible. Neuropathy and encephalopathy may also follow acute poisoning.

Differential diagnosis

In acute poisoning, other causes of similar clinical manifestations must be excluded, such as respiratory diseases, acute diarrhoeal diseases, and affections of the central nervous and cardiovascular systems. The inhibition of blood cholinesterase activity and a history of exposure to organophosphorus pesticides are important diagnostic indicators. The diagnosis of chronic poisoning is extremely difficult. If other causes of ill health have been excluded, high-level persistent exposure to organophosphorus pesticides may be assumed to be the causative factor.

Susceptibility

Individuals with a physiologically low level of blood cholinesterase are supposed to be more susceptible to organophosphorus poisoning. However, this assumption has not been confirmed. Diseases of the nervous system, liver, and kidney (impairment of biotransformation and/or excretion) may increase susceptibility.

Health examinations

Preplacement examination

The preplacement examination should include a medical history and a physical examination, with special attention to the nervous and respiratory systems, liver, and kidneys. Blood cholinesterase activity should also be measured.

Periodic examinations

In medical terms the periodic examination is the same as the preplacement one. It should be carried out at intervals depending on the nature of the work and on the toxicity of the substance in question. In regular long-term exposure (e.g., that resulting from the production or formulation of pesticides), intervals of several months may be necessary, otherwise it may be sufficient to do the examination annually.

Screening test

Blood cholinesterase activity should be measured, particularly in spraymen, immediately following the period of high exposure. The inhibition of the activity of blood cholinesterase by 25% in comparison with the pre-exposure value is considered statistically significant since it exceeds laboratory error.

Case management

In acute poisoning, remove the patient from further exposure. If there has been any skin contact with an organophosphorus compound, wash the affected area with soap and warm water. In patients showing parasympathetic nervous system stimulation, administer atropine by mouth or, in more severe cases, by injection. Symptoms involving the central and autonomic nervous systems should be treated with sedatives (barbiturates). Other symptoms such as vomiting, diarrhoea, and chest tightness should be treated accordingly. Resuscitation may also be necessary. Oximes act as cholinesterase reactivators.

The inhibition of cholinesterase activity may also be found in asymptomatic workers. There is disagreement among experts regarding the level of cholinesterase inhibition at which further exposure should be avoided. While some experts recommend temporary removal of workers from exposure when 25% of the cholinesterase activity is found to be inhibited, others believe that removal from further exposure need not take place as long as the inhibition level is below 50%.

Patients with chronic poisoning should be permanently removed from further exposure.

Control measures

Technical control measures should be taken to reduce exposure levels. However, good work practice and the use of personal protective devices (overalls, gloves, respirators) are extremely effective ways of preventing exposure.

It is impracticable to summarize exposure limits expressed as air concentrations because of the great variety of compounds involved. A WHO Study Group has recommended that the inhibition of cholinesterase activity by 30% of the pre-exposure level should be regarded as a biological exposure limit.[1]

---

[1] WHO Technical Report Series, No. 677, 1982.

CHAPTER 10

Diseases caused by chromium and its toxic compounds

Properties of the causal agents

Chromium is a hard whitish metal with a melting point of 1890 °C. Chromium(II) compounds are relatively unstable and oxidize readily to the stable chromium(III) state. Hexavalent chromium salts are strong oxidizing compounds and are easily reduced to the trivalent state.

Occurrence and uses

The most common chromium ore is ferrous chromite ($FeCr_2O_3$). Chromium and its compounds are encountered particularly in metallurgical and chemical industries, e.g., in the production and use of chromium pigments, in leather tanning and chromium plating industries, and in the manufacture of chromium alloys and stainless steel. Small amounts of chromium are present in most types of cement.

Occupations involving risk of chromium exposure

Workers in industries producing mono- and dichromate and ferrochromium alloys, stainless steel welders, chromium platers, furniture polishers, chromium pigment spray painters, leather tanners and other leather workers, cement producers and building workers, printers, and photographic technicians are at greatest risk of exposure. Up to 80–90 different occupations are thought to carry some risk of exposure to chromium and its compounds.

Mechanism of action

Absorption

Although the lungs are considered to be the most important route of entry in occupational exposure, information on the uptake of chromium from the lungs is fragmentary. The mechanisms of deposition and retention of chromium dust and fumes in the lungs appear to be the same as those of other dusts and aerosols.

Trivalent chromium compounds are generally absorbed in the body to a much lesser extent than the hexavalent compounds. Depending on the solubility of the compound, 0.2–3% of trivalent compounds and 1–10% of hexavalent compounds that enter the body via the oral route are absorbed.

Chromium pigment particles, chromium fumes from stainless steel welding, and chromic acid mist aerosols consist of particles generally smaller than 1 μm, resulting in maximum alveolar penetration.[1] Higher water solubility considerably increases the uptake and toxicity of chromium compounds.

Biotransformation

Hexavalent chromium compounds are reduced to the trivalent state in the body. The rate of reduction depends on the amount of reducing agents in the exposed organs, and this influences the toxicity and excretion of the hexavalent compounds.

Excretion

Excretion takes place mainly through the urine and faeces. The rate of excretion varies considerably for different chromium compounds.

Assessment of exposure

Environmental assessment

The measurement of atmospheric concentration of chromium is the most reliable method of assessing exposure. When collecting hexavalent compounds on filters, the possibility of their reduction to the trivalent state before analysis should be taken into account. Both the respirable fraction and the total concentration should be determined. This is important particularly for aerosols with low water solubility (such as chromium carbonate, lead or zinc chromate, and welding fumes), the larger particles of which are cleared from the respiratory tract without absorption. So far as highly soluble chromium compounds are concerned (e.g., chromium acetate, chromium trioxide (chromic acid), and potassium and sodium chromate or dichromate), all particle sizes are of toxicological concern, since large particles deposited in the upper airways dissolve and may be absorbed.

---

[1] Maximum alveolar penetration occurs with particles of approximately 1 μm diameter and below. However, the deposition in the pulmonary spaces, which is almost 100% for particles of 2 μm, decreases with particle size below this value and reaches a minimum for particles of about 0.5 μm.

Biological assessment

Attempts to relate urinary concentrations of chromium to the concentration of chromium in the working atmosphere have not produced any reliable criteria for the determination of exposure level. The determination of chromium concentration in plasma or whole-blood within 24 hours after a single accidental oral intake and after short-term inhalation exposure to high concentrations of chromates may be of some help in determining the dose or exposure level. The determination of chromium concentration in erythrocytes may be a useful indicator of exposure even up to 7–8 weeks after a single high-dose exposure.

Clinical effects

There is no evidence that the most important chromium-containing ore (chromite) or chromium metal is toxic to man. The trivalent chromium compounds are generally much less toxic than the hexavalent ones.

Acute effects

Accidental ingestion of hexavalent chromium compounds may cause bleeding in the gastrointestinal tract, necrosis of the liver, or tubular necrosis of the kidneys.

Chronic effects

The local deposition of chromates on mucous membranes may cause ulcerations in the nasal septum, which quite often leads to perforation. Ulcers in the throat and in the upper airways have also been reported. The deposition of chromates on the skin may lead to deep ulceration ("chrome holes"), particularly at the finger-roots and on the finger-knuckles, but also at other sites where chromates have been deposited without proper washing afterwards.

Skin allergy to chromates is probably the most common untoward health effect. It is reported to be the cause of contact dermatitis in up to 13% of male cases. A skin patch test with low concentrations of potassium chromate is the most commonly used method for confirming the diagnosis. Trivalent chromium compounds are also capable of eliciting an allergic reaction to chromium.

An asthmatic reaction has been reported in workers exposed to chromic acid and chromate aerosols and in stainless steel welders exposed to chromium and nickel compounds through welding fumes.

Delayed effects

It has been established that hexavalent chromium compounds are carcinogenic. A higher than average incidence of bronchogenic cancer has been demonstrated in workers exposed to dichromate and chromium pigments. There is some weak evidence of increased cancer incidence in painters, users of chromium pigments, workers exposed to chromic acid mist, stainless steel welders, and in those employed in the production of ferrochromium alloys.

Exposure–effect relationship

Serious acute poisoning develops after ingestion of 1–9 g of hexavalent chromium compounds. Damage to mucous membranes was found after exposure to chromic acid fumes at atmospheric concentrations of about 0.1 mg/m^3 and higher, but no information is available on the effects of particles of Cr^{6+} at lower concentrations. The exposure–effect relationship for lung cancer is not yet established.

Prognosis

Recovery from skin and mucous membrane ulcerations and even allergic dermatitis may be complete if exposure to chromium compounds is discontinued. However, skin allergy may persist and later contact with trace amounts of chromium (e.g., chromium-tanned leather wear) may cause relapse. The perforation of nasal septum and atrophic rhinitis are irreversible conditions. The prognosis of chromium-associated lung cancer does not differ from that of lung cancers of other etiologies.

Differential diagnosis

Ulcers and perforation of the nasal septum are also caused by corrosive metals and compounds other than chromium. Therefore, in order to ascertain the exact etiology of such conditions, a documented occupational history is essential. Ulcers caused by exposure to chromium are quite easy to differentiate from other similar skin conditions: the typical chromium ulcers are deep and round and have elevated margins.

Skin patch tests are important in differentiating allergic dermatitis due to chromium exposure from other allergic skin reactions. Also, provocation tests have been used for demonstrating asthma due to chromium exposure. However, it should be noted that evidence of occupational exposure to chromium is indispensable for confirming the diagnosis in both cases.

Lung cancer cases in chromate workers are most frequently of the epithelial type and do not differ histologically from other lung cancers caused by environmental carcinogens.

Susceptibility

Persons with a previous history of asthmatic reaction to air-borne chromates or of skin reaction to chromates or other chromium compounds are more susceptible than others. Such workers should be advised not to take up jobs involving exposure to chromium and its compounds. Whether or not cross-reactions to other allergens occur is not known. However, it seems advisable not to employ atopic subjects in jobs involving a considerable risk of inhalation exposure or of skin exposure to chromium compounds.

Potentiation of exposure to chromates by tobacco smoke has been postulated, but the evidence is still weak.

Health examinations

Preplacement examination

The preplacement examination should include a medical history and a physical examination, with special attention to allergies and respiratory and skin diseases.

Periodic examinations

In medical terms the periodic examination is the same as the preplacement one. It should be carried out at one year intervals. In addition, rhinoscopy should be done.

Screening tests

For the early detection of lung cancer in heavily exposed workers, screening by means of chest X-ray and sputum cytology in workers at greatest risk has been suggested, but the absence of effective treatment and difficulties in cytological interpretation seriously limit the value of this approach.

Case management

In cases of accidental ingestion of chromates, milk as first aid and reducing agents such as ascorbic acid should be given immediately. The quick reduction of Cr^{6+} into Cr^{3+} is most important. In cases of skin allergy and asthma, a change to different work seems generally advisable. In the initial phase of ulcer development, local application of reducing agents at the site of ulceration may limit progression. Lung cancer cases should be treated in the same way as lung cancers of other etiologies.

Control measures

Technical control measures should be taken to reduce the concentration of chromium in the workroom air. In order to prevent skin contact, personal protective devices (particularly gloves, clothes, protective creams) should be used wherever necessary. Good personal hygiene, i.e., regular washing of hands, taking a shower after the workshift, and the use of regenerative skin creams, is very important.

The exposure limits for chromic compounds vary in different countries from $0.01\,mg(Cr)/m^3$ to $0.1\,mg(Cr)/m^3$; for chromium and its insoluble compounds, the exposure limits range from $0.5\,mg/m^3$ to $1\,mg/m^3$.

Since chromates are carcinogenic, exposure should be kept as low as possible.

CHAPTER 11

Diseases caused by manganese and its toxic compounds

Properties of the causal agent

Manganese is a whitish-grey brittle metal that exists in eight oxidation states. Manganese dioxide (MnO_2) is the most stable oxide. Among organometallic compounds, manganese 2-methylcyclopenta-dienyl tricarbonyl (MMT) and manganese cyclopentadienyl tricarbonyl (CMT) are most important.

Occurrence and uses

Manganese oxides, carbonates, and silicates are the most important among the manganese-containing minerals, the most common ore being MnO_2 (pyrolusite), which is usually mined by opencast techniques.

About 90% of all the manganese mined in the world is used in the steel industry as a reagent to reduce oxygen and sulfur. Other major uses are: in the production of dry cell batteries; and in the production of potassium permanganate and other manganese compounds. Manganese is also used in electrode coating of welding rods. Certain of its compounds are used as driers for linseed oil, glass and textile bleaching, dyeing, tanning of leather, and the manufacture of ferti-lizers. Organic carbonyl compounds of manganese are used as addi-tives in fuel oil, smoke inhibitors, and as antiknock additives in petrol.

Occupations involving risk of exposure to manganese

Manganese miners, workers in the ferromanganese and iron and steel industries, and those involved in the production of dry cell batteries and welding rods are at greatest risk.

Mechanism of action

Absorption

Manganese and its compounds enter the body mainly by inhalation. Since most manganese compounds are practically insoluble in water, only particles small enough to reach the alveoli are eventually absorbed. Manganese may also enter the gastrointestinal tract with contaminated food and water; about 3% of ingested manganese is absorbed.

Distribution

The absorbed manganese is rapidly cleared from the blood and distributed to other tissues, mainly the liver. It can cross the blood–brain barrier and may also pass through the placenta. Manganese is an essential metalloprotein component of some enzymes.

Excretion

The biological half-life of manganese is about 40 days, but for manganese in the brain it is considerably longer than for the whole body. The bile flow is the most important route of excretion. Thus, it is eliminated almost entirely with the faeces and only about 0.1–1.3% of the daily intake is excreted in the urine. After exposure to MMT, however, the excretion of manganese in the urine is much greater, reaching about 30% of the total amount.

Assessment of exposure

Environmental assessment

Periodic measurements of manganese concentrations in the workroom air (both total dust and respirable fraction) should be performed, preferably by personal sampling. However, the correlation between air concentration and the degree of health damage to the worker is rather weak.

Biological assessment

The determination of manganese in urine and blood is not of great value. The mean concentration in the urine on a group basis correlates roughly with the mean air concentration, but in individuals the correlation is poor. In persons not occupationally exposed to manganese, the concentration of manganese does not exceed 20 µg/litre in blood, 2 µg/litre in urine, and 3 mg/kg in hair. A manganese concentration of 60 mg/kg in the faeces has been suggested as indicative of occupational exposure to manganese.

Clinical effects

Acute effects

Acute poisoning by manganese compounds occurs only rarely as the consequence of an accident.

Chronic effects

Long-term exposure to manganese causes damage to the central nervous system and lungs.

Effects on the central nervous system (manganism). The first sign of manganese poisoning is impaired mental capacity. It may result from exposure to high concentrations of manganese dusts or fumes for only a few months or even less. Usually it appears after a prolonged exposure of two or more years. Disorders of the central nervous system are accompanied by many other symptoms. In its course, the disease can be divided into three phases:

(*a*) a subclinical stage with generally vague symptomatology;

(*b*) an early clinical stage in which psychic or neurological symptoms and signs predominate and include acute psychomotor disturbances, dysarthria, and disturbance of gait; and

(*c*) a fully developed stage associated with manic or depressive psychosis and parkinsonism.

Effects on the lungs. An increased incidence of pneumonia as well as a higher rate of acute and chronic bronchitis (particularly if the exposure is combined with smoking) have been reported in exposure to high concentrations of manganese in the air. Manganese seems to decrease immunological resistance to respiratory bacterial or viral infections.

Other reported effects of manganese include: decreased blood pressure, dysproteinaemia, and reproductive disturbances. However, these effects have not been conclusively demonstrated.

Exposure–effect relationship

Adverse effects on the central nervous system have been reported at manganese concentrations of 2–5 mg/m^3 of air. Nonspecific symptoms and signs may appear at a concentration of about 0.5 mg manganese/m^3 of air. Adverse effects on the lungs have not been reported at concentrations below 0.3–0.5 mg/m^3 of air.

Prognosis

If the worker is removed from exposure shortly after the onset of the symptoms and signs, partial reversal may take place. However, some residual disturbances, particularly in speech and gait may persist. In the developed stage of manganism, disability is permanent.

Differential diagnosis

Other causes of nonspecific symptoms and signs should be excluded. An occupational history of exposure to manganese is essential.

Susceptibility

Pregnant women may run the risk of abortion following exposure to manganese. Persons suffering from chronic infections, liver and kidney diseases (decreased elimination of manganese), nutritional deficiency and iron-deficiency anaemia (increased absorption of manganese), and chronic obstructive pulmonary disease are at greatest risk. Alcoholics and smokers also run a higher than average risk of developing manganese-related diseases. Persons with psychic or neurological disorders should be advised not to work with manganese.

Health examinations

Preplacement examination

The preplacement examination should include medical history and a physical examination with special attention to the nervous and respiratory systems.

Periodic examinations

In medical terms the periodic examination is the same as the preplacement one. Periodic examinations may be required once a year or less often, depending on the level of exposure encountered in the job. Special emphasis should be given to behavioural and neurological disturbances such as: speech defects, emotional disturbances, tremor, impairment of equilibrium, difficulty in walking or squatting, adiadochokinesia, and disturbances in handwriting. Subjective symptoms and abnormal behaviour may often constitute the only early indications of health impairment.

Case management

Workers suffering from manganism should be removed from further exposure to manganese. Treatment with orally administered levodopa has been recommended.

Control measures

A primary control measure should be the suppression of manganese dusts and fumes. Dry drilling in mines should always be replaced by wet drilling. Airline respiratory protection equipment as well as independent respirators should be used to avoid high-level short-term exposure. A high standard of personal hygiene is essential. Showering and changing of clothes after work should be made compulsory and there should be a ban on eating and smoking at the workplace.

Exposure limits for manganese in different countries range from 0.3 mg/m³ to 6 mg/m³. A WHO Study Group[1] has recommended a health-based exposure limit of 0.3 mg of respirable manganese particles per cubic metre of air (time-weighted average) for occupational exposure.

[1] WHO Technical Report Series, No. 647, 1980.

CHAPTER 12

Diseases caused by arsenic and its toxic compounds

Properties of the causal agents

Elemental arsenic is a silvery lustrous metalloid. When heated, it sublimes without melting. Arsenic compounds (arsenic(III) oxide, arsenic(V) oxide, the acids formed from these oxides and their salts, and organic arsenic compounds) are more commonly encountered than arsenic metal.

Occurrence and uses

Arsenic is found in iron ore and coal, and is widely distributed in nature in small amounts. It is also found in traces (less than 1 mg/kg) in most living organisms, including those man uses for food.

Arsenic trioxide is used in the synthesis of many other arsenic compounds. Some arsenates are used as pesticides. Various arsenic compounds are used as wood preservatives, animal feed additives, and as agents in the production of glass, lead alloys, drugs, and semiconductors.

Occupations involving risk of exposure to arsenic

Agriculture and forestry workers who apply arsenic pesticides, workers in arsenic refineries and ore smelters, those involved in the manufacture of wood preservatives, pesticides, and drugs, and metallurgy and electronics industry workers are at greatest risk. Arsine gas is used in the lacquer industry.

Mechanism of action

Absorption

Arsenic dust and fumes enter the body through inhalation. Absorption from skin may occur when arsenic compounds come into contact with open abrasions. Arsenic acids may be absorbed through intact skin.

Arsenic particles encountered in the workplace are relatively large, and therefore they deposit primarily in the upper respiratory passages—i.e., from the nose to the bronchi. Some particles, however, reach the lower regions of the lungs, from where they are absorbed. Absorption also takes place in the gastrointestinal tract when the particles cleared from the upper respiratory tract are swallowed.

Biotransformation

Trivalent arsenic may be oxidized in the body to the pentavalent state. The opposite can also take place. Inorganic arsenic is methylated to form dimethylarsinic acid and methylarsonic acid. Arsenic may be organically bound to sulfhydryl groups.

Excretion

Most of the absorbed arsenic is excreted in the urine, with small amounts being excreted in the faeces. The maximum excretion occurs in the first 6 hours, with about 25 % being excreted in 24 hours and about 75 % within 7 days of exposure.

Assessment of exposure

Environmental assessment

Regular monitoring by personal sampling is the method of choice. If this is not possible for some reason, area sampling, preferably in the breathing zone, should be done.

Biological assessment

Arsenic is best determined in the urine. In subjects not occupationally exposed to arsenic, the concentration of arsenic in the urine does not usually exceed 30 µg/litre. Seafood dramatically increases the concentration of arsenic in the urine. Therefore, seafood must be avoided at least two days before urine sampling. A concentration of arsenic in the urine of 1000 µg/litre corresponds roughly to a time-weighted average concentration of arsenic in air of 250 µg/m³. For the determination of past exposure, analysis of arsenic in hair may be useful.

Clinical effects

Acute poisoning

Acute poisoning occurs only from the ingestion of arsenic compounds. The symptoms of acute poisoning include: severe vomiting and diarrhoea, muscular cramps, facial oedema, and cardiac abnormalities. Shock is possible, and dehydration frequently follows. The fatal dose of ingested elemental arsenic is in the range 70–180 mg. When high concentrations of airborne inorganic arsenic compounds are inhaled, inflammation of the upper respiratory tract may occur (rhinitis, pharyngitis, laryngitis).

Skin changes following contact with arsenic compounds include: contact dermatitis, folliculitis, eczematous eruptions, and ulcerations.

In the presence of nascent hydrogen, arsenic can unite with the hydrogen ion and form arsine (AsH_3), which is an odourless, colourless gas slightly irritating to the nasopharynx. It is absorbed from the lungs into the blood and causes haemolysis of the red blood cells. In about 6 hours, severe haemoglobinuria occurs. Heavy arsine exposure, if untreated, may cause the haemoglobin to precipitate in the kidney tubules, causing lower nephron nephritis with complete loss of kidney function.

Chronic poisoning

In long-term exposure, arsenic can affect the skin, respiratory tract, heart, liver, kidneys, blood and blood-producing organs, and the nervous system. Skin changes include: increased pigmentation, herpetic lesions about the mouth, furfuraceous desquamation,[1] hyperkeratoses (especially of the palms and soles), and, in rare cases, skin cancer. Perforation of the nasal septum may develop and so may chronic bronchitis, and possibly, increased basilar fibrosis of the lungs. Neither liver nor kidney damage is common, though occasionally cirrhosis of the liver may develop. Vascular lesions (endangiitis obliterans, acrodermatitis) have been reported on rare occasions. An increased mortality from cardiovascular diseases has been reported in two epidemiological investigations. Reversible damage to the peripheral nerves follows subacute exposure, and recovery is often slow. These neurological deficits are frequently subclinical and are not discernible by clinical neurological tests; however, they can be detected by measuring nerve conduction velocity and by electromyography. Chronic exposure to arsenic compounds can affect haematopoiesis (normochromic anaemia, neutropenia, thrombocytopenia).

Delayed effects

Exposure to arsenic has been associated with pulmonary cancer in several occupations. A relationship between leukaemia, lymphomas, and arsenic exposure has been reported, but the evidence is not conclusive.

Exposure–effect relationship

Irritation of the skin and mucous membranes is less probable at air concentrations of arsenic below 0.5 mg/m³. Although data are

---

[1] The shedding of epithelial elements of the skin in bran-like scales.

uncertain, it has been estimated that exposure to airborne arsenic concentrations of about 50 μg/m^3 for more than 25 years would result in a nearly 3-fold increase in mortality due to lung cancer over the age of 65 years.

Prognosis

The prognosis of irritating effects of arsenic is excellent. Permanent damage to the heart, lungs, liver, and nervous system are rare in industrial exposures. However, mortality from bronchiogenic cancer is extremely high.

Differential diagnosis

In acute poisoning, exclude other causes of acute gastroenteritis and respiratory tract and skin irritation. The presence of arsenic in a high concentration is an important factor in diagnosis. In chronic poisoning, a well documented history of exposure to arsenic compounds is essential. Other causes of chronic respiratory disease, neurological disease, hepatitis, nephritis, and lung cancer should be excluded.

Susceptibility

There are no known factors that increase susceptibility. Pregnant women may be at an increased risk of having abnormal fetuses, but the data are not conclusive. Increased arsenic body burden, from both occupational or non-occupational sources may be regarded as a risk factor.

Health examinations

Preplacement examination

The preplacement examination should include a medical history, a physical examination, and a chest X-ray. An examination of the nasal passages and skin should also be carried out.

Periodic examination

In medical terms, the periodic examination is the same as the preplacement one. In addition, liver and kidney function tests should be done. The periodic examination should be repeated once every year.

After ten years of continuous exposure to arsenic and its compounds, chest X-rays should be taken at intervals depending on the worker's age and level of exposure; one-year intervals are usually recommended. Sputum cytology examinations are of questionable value.

The principal purpose of the periodic examination is to ensure that the person does not develop chronic skin or respiratory problems and to detect early the development of bronchiogenic cancer.

Screening test

In workplaces with high arsenic air concentrations, it is desirable to carry out urine analysis for arsenic every 3 months. If this is not possible, a urine analysis should be done at least annually.

Case management

If the concentration of arsenic in the urine of one worker indicates excessive exposure, the urine of that worker should be retested and urine analysis should be done in others performing similar work. If the concentration remains elevated, industrial hygiene and personal hygiene practices should be revised and appropriate steps should be taken to reduce exposure. Acute arsenic poisoning responds well to treatment with dimercaprol. Persons with chronic poisoning should be removed from exposure. Although dimercaprol is generally not effective in chronic exposure, in some individuals it may give positive results.

Heavy arsine exposure should be treated by total blood transfusion.

Control measures

Since arsenic is a carcinogen (or a co-carcinogen), all efforts should be made to reduce exposure to the minimum possible level. The use of enclosed systems (as far as possible), local ventilation, and personal protective devices against skin contact or respiratory absorption are recommended.

The exposure limits in different countries range from $0.05 \, \mu g/m^3$ to $0.5 \, \mu g/m^3$ for arsenic, and 0.05 to $0.4 \, \mu g/m^3$ for arsine.

CHAPTER 13

Diseases caused by mercury and its toxic compounds

Properties of the causal agents

Mercury is a silvery liquid metal with a melting point of $-39\,°C$. It evaporates at room temperature. It forms a variety of compounds, both inorganic (such as oxides, sulfates, chlorides, and nitrates) and organic (alkyl and aryl). Mercury compounds of low solubility in water usually have low toxicity.

Occurrence and uses

The most important ore of mercury is cinnabar (HgS). Metallic mercury is used in the electrolytic production of sodium and potassium hydroxides and chlorine as well as in the manufacture and repair of measurement or laboratory equipment (barometers, thermometers, etc.); in the manufacture of mercury vapour tubes, X-ray tubes, rectifiers, etc.; and in the production of amalgams.

Mercury(II) chloride ($HgCl_2$), used at one time as a disinfectant, is now used as a fungicide (usually mixed with mercury(I) chloride, Hg_2Cl_2) for treating bulbs and protecting wood. Aryl and alkyl mercury compounds are used in agriculture as fungicides or as disinfectants. Methylmercury (alkyl) is very toxic and should not be used. Akyl mercury compounds are formed in the environment naturally by the methylation of mercury by microplankton in the sea. They are deposited in sea animals, mainly in fish and molluscs, and reach man via such seafoods.

Occupations involving risk of mercury exposure

The main hazard arises from occupational exposure to the vapours of elemental mercury. This type of exposure is encountered in: mercury-ore mining; production of metallic mercury in metallurgy; production of sodium and potassium hydroxides, dyes, fluorescent lamps; production and repair of electrical measuring devices, laboratory instruments; amalgam production in dentistry; and seed treatment and wood protection by organic compounds of mercury. There are many more occupations with potential exposure to mercury.

Mechanism of action

Absorption

Mercury enters the body mainly through the lungs as vapour or dust. About 80% of the inhaled mercury vapours are absorbed. Ingested metallic mercury is absorbed from the digestive tract only in small, negligible amounts, whereas water-soluble mercury compounds are readily absorbed. Some organic and inorganic mercury(II) compounds may be absorbed through the skin. The daily intake of mercury with food is in the range of a few micrograms.

Biotransformation

Absorbed elemental mercury is quickly oxidized to the Hg^{2+} ion, which has an affinity with sulfhydryl (-SH) groups, and binds to substrates rich in them. The highest concentration of mercury is found in the kidneys (bound to metallothionein) and liver. Mercury is able to pass through the blood–brain barrier and the placenta. Methylmercury has a strong affinity with the brain. About 90% of mercury in blood is found in the erythrocytes. The metabolism of the aryl compounds of mercury is similar to that of metallic mercury or of inorganic compounds. The phenyl and methoxyethyl compounds of mercury are rapidly converted into inorganic mercury, whereas methylated mercury is metabolized very slowly.

Excretion

While elemental mercury and its inorganic compounds are eliminated more in urine than in faeces, organic compounds are mainly excreted in the faeces (up to 90%). The biological half-life of inorganic mercury is approximately 6 weeks.

Assessment of exposure

Environmental assessment

Air samples can be analysed by atomic absorption spectrometry or dithisone colorimetry. Portable devices that measure the absorption of light emitted by the mercury discharge lamp are also used.

Biological assesssment

The best method of assessing exposure to mercury vapours and inorganic or aryl compounds of mercury is the determination of mercury quantitatively in the urine by atomic absorption spectrometry or dithisone colorimetry. In exposure to organic compounds (methylmercury), the concentration of these compounds in the erythrocytes and plasma should be measured.

In subjects not occupationally exposed to mercury, the urine concentration of mercury is less than 20 µg/litre. There seems to be a linear relationship between the concentration of mercury in air and its concentration in the urine. In the literature, the ratio between air concentration and the concentration in urine is given variously as 1:2 to 1:3. According to one estimate, the average air concentration of mercury of 50 µg/m³ corresponds to a concentration in urine of 100–150 µg/litre. There is, however, great individual variation in both the correlation between exposure level and excretion level and in the amount of mercury excreted each day.

Clinical effects

Exposure to inorganic mercury vapour may damage the nervous system. Methylmercury is extremely toxic to the nervous system, whereas phenyl and methoxyethyl compounds are of low toxicity.

Acute poisoning

Short-term exposure to metallic mercury vapour in concentrations of several mg/m³ of air causes irritation of the bronchial mucous membranes, stomatitis with increased salivation, and pneumonitis accompanied by fever and dyspnoea. Accidental ingestion of inorganic salts such as mercury(II) chloride ($HgCl_2$), causes local necrosis in the mouth and digestive tract, circulatory collapse, and acute failure of kidneys, with oliguria and anuria.

Chronic poisoning

The classical triad described in chronic poisoning due to mercury vapour comprises erethism, tremor, and stomatitis. Neurological and psychic symptoms are the most characteristic. Nonspecific early symptoms (anorexia, weight loss, headaches) are followed by more characteristic disorders: increased irritability, sleep disturbances (frequent waking, insomnia), excitability, anxiety, depression, memory defects, and loss of self-confidence. Problems of a more serious nature, such as hallucinations, complete loss of memory, and deterioration of intellectual ability, are not seen nowadays. Mercurial tremor is of the mixed type (i.e., both persistent and intention tremor are present) and may be seen at first as fine tremor of closed eyelids, lips and tongue, and fingers. The handwriting becomes shaky, irregular, and often illegible. The tremor progresses, affecting the arms and eventually the whole body. Severe poisoning often results in speech defects, especially affecting pronunciation. Other neurological signs include flushing, increased perspiration, and dermatographia. Chronic gingivitis often occurs and may lead to the loss of teeth. In spite of the high degree of mercury accumulation in the kidneys, renal damage is rare. Mercury deposits in the anterior capsule of the crystalline lens of the eye causing a grey-brown or yellow reflex from the lens.

Occupational poisonings with aryl (phenyl) and methoxyethyl organic compounds of mercury are very rare. Their effects are similar to those caused by inorganic mercury because of their rapid transformation in the body to this form. In addition, they may cause toxic dermatitis.

Delayed effects

There is no evidence of cancerogenicity of inorganic mercury. However, some experimental studies have reported chromosomal and mitotic aberrations as a consequence of exposure to mercury.

Exposure–effects relationship

Acute pulmonary effects occur at exposure to concentrations of mercury vapour in the range of $1-3 \text{ mg/m}^3$. Concentrations of metallic and inorganic mercury of 0.05 mg/m^3 and less are not believed to lead to intoxication in workers exposed for 8 hours daily for 5 days a week.

Prognosis

The prognosis of chronic intoxication is good once exposure has ceased, particularly if the intoxication is not allowed to progress beyond the early stages.

Differential diagnosis

Acute poisoning

Acute bronchitis, interstitial pneumonitis, and stomatitis of mercurial origin are confirmed by a relevant work history, evidence of occupational exposure to high concentrations of mercury in air, and the presence of mercury in high concentrations in the urine.

Chronic poisoning

Mercurial tremor is similar to the tremors seen in multiple sclerosis, certain muscular diseases, and alcoholism. Sometimes it is difficult to distinguish mental changes (referred to as erethism) from other exogenous neuroses and some other diseases. A history of occupational exposure to mercury and the presence of high concentrations of mercury in the urine help to confirm or exclude the mercurial etiology of tremors and mental changes.

Susceptibility

Adolescents, pregnant women, lactating mothers, and those suffering from organic or functional neurological and mental diseases, diseases of kidney parenchyma and liver, hyperthyroidism, or chronic alcoholism are at greatest risk.

Health examinations

Preplacement examination

The preplacement examination should include a medical history and a physical examination, with special attention to the oral cavity, nervous system, and mental health. A sample of handwriting should be taken and filed for future reference.

Periodic examination

In medical terms, the periodic examination is the same as the preplacement one. Depending on the level of exposure, it may be carried out at intervals of 6–12 months. If the exposure is very high, it may be necessary to repeat the examination at even shorter intervals.

In order to detect mercurial tremor, a sample of handwriting should be checked against the reference sample taken at the preplacement examination. In workplaces involving exposure to organic compounds of mercury, an ophthalmological examination of the visual field should also be done.

Case management

At the first appearance of symptoms of mercury poisoning, remove the worker from further exposure and keep him away at least until the symptoms and signs disappear. Symptom-free workers with a concentration of mercury in the urine exceeding 100 µg/litre should also be kept away from exposure until the concentration drops below that level. If some signs and symptoms persist after long-term (several years) exposure, the worker should be permanently removed from mercury exposure. The efficacy of treatment with dimercaprol (2,3 dimercaptopropanol), unithiol (sodium 2,3-dimercapto-1-propane sulfonate), or penicillamine is questionable.

Control measures

Whenever possible, mercury should be handled in hermetically sealed systems and strict hygiene should be enforced at workplaces.

Moreover, it is essential to prevent: (a) the escape of mercury from containers; (b) the dispersion of its droplets in the air; and (c) the infiltration of mercury into crevices and gaps in the floors or working tables (this causes long-lasting evaporation). Mercury vapour and dust containing mercury compounds should be suppressed by technical control measures. In emergencies involving exposure to high mercury vapour concentrations, protective respiratory devices should be worn.

The exposure limits for elemental mercury vary in different countries from $0.01 \, mg/m^3$ to $0.05 \, mg/m^3$. The health-based exposure limit recommended by a WHO Study Group is $25 \, \mu g/m^3$ in air (time-weighted average) or $50 \, \mu g/g$ creatinine in urine.[1]

---

[1] WHO Technical Report Series, No. 647, 1980.

CHAPTER 14

Diseases caused by lead and its toxic compounds

Properties of the causal agent

Lead is a bluish-grey heavy metal with melting and boiling points of 327 °C and 1620 °C, respectively. At a temperature of 550–600 °C, lead evaporates and combines with oxygen in the air to form lead oxide. Its most common oxidation state is lead(II) and the most important organometallic compounds are lead tetraethyl, lead tetramethyl, and lead stearate.

Occurrence and uses

Lead is universally present in small amounts in rocks, soil, and plants. The principal lead ore is galena (PbS), which is usually found associated with sulfides of silver, copper, arsenic, antimony, bismuth, and tin. Other common lead ores are cerussite ($PbCO_3$) and anglesite ($PbSO_4$). Lead is commercially produced by mining, smelting, refining, and secondary recovery.

Metallic lead is used in: shielding electrical cables; production of pipes, cisterns, roof coverings; sealing joints; coating metals exposed to the weather, especially to sea water (red lead); manufacture of lead-acid storage batteries (accumulator plates); the chemical industry for lining containers for sulfuric acid, evaporation pans, etc; the manufacture of various alloys with tin, copper, and antimony in the printing and ammunitions industries; the production of lead pigments for paints and varnishes; and the manufacture of flint glass and vitreous enamelling. Lead-glazed earthenware and flaking lead paints in old houses are other possible sources of lead exposure in the domestic environment. Lead alkyls (tetraethyl lead, tetramethyl lead) are used in the petroleum industry as antiknock additives in fuels.

Occupations involving risk of lead exposure

Workers in smelting and storage battery manufacturing plants, scrap workers, painters, potters, workers in the ceramics industry, foundry workers, welders, and petrol blenders, are among those at greatest risk of exposure.

Mechanism of action

Absorption

Lead and its compounds enter the body by inhalation and ingestion. Absorption through the skin is of importance only in the case of organic compounds (lead alkyls and lead naphthenates).

Lead intake in the general population is estimated to be between 100 µg/day and 350 µg/day. Although the main sources are food and water, as much as 20 µg may be absorbed from the inhalation of lead vapour and particulate matter in polluted urban environments.

The hazard to health from airborne lead is related to its particle size. Particles smaller than 10 µm can be retained in the lungs, whereas larger particles are deposited in the upper respiratory tract, from where they are transported by the mucociliary movement to the nasopharynx, and swallowed. On average 10–30% of the inhaled lead is absorbed through the lungs, and about 5–10% of the ingested lead is absorbed through the gastrointestinal tract. Tetraethyl lead vapour is well absorbed through the lungs.

Distribution

The absorbed lead is transported by the blood to other organs. About 95% of blood lead is bound to the red blood cells. A fraction of plasma lead is in the diffusible form, supposedly in equilibrium with other body pools of lead, which may be divided into two: hard tissues (bones, hair, nails, teeth); and soft tissues (bone marrow, nervous system, kidneys, liver). It is thought that only lead in soft tissues is directly toxic. Lead in hard tissues remains tightly bound to the tissues and is toxic only when the pool serves as a source of soft tissue lead. Owing to the distribution of lead between hard and soft tissues, the biological half-life of lead is difficult to establish. However, there is no doubt that clearance of half the body burden of lead would require a number of years.

Excretion

Lead is excreted via both urine (75–80%) and faeces (about 15%). Even after moderate absorption, lead appears quickly in the urine. It seems that the body reaches an equilibrium between absorption and excretion in which the amount of lead excreted in urine, faeces, bile, sweat, hair, and nails corresponds to the amount absorbed. The process of renal clearance of lead is essentially glomerular filtration. The rate of biliary excretion of lead in man is not known.

Assessment of exposure

Environmental assessment

In occupational settings, regular fixed-station air monitoring at carefully chosen sites and the measurement of individual exposure by personal samplers can provide useful information. However, the monitoring of exposure by biological means in individual workers offers several advantages over air monitoring.

Biological assessment

There are two kinds of biological test: (*a*) those that determine the presence of lead in blood and urine; and (*b*) those that measure the biochemical and haematological toxic effects of lead. Among the latter, the biochemical tests include the measurement of: the activity of delta-aminolevulinate dehydratase (ALAD) in blood; the amount of delta-aminolevulinic acid (δ-ALA) in urine; the amount of coproporphyrin in urine; and the concentration of zinc protoporphyrin IX (ZnPP) in red blood cells.

The haematological tests are based on the determination of the extent of blood damage due to lead exposure. Increased lead absorption leads to: (*a*) decreased content of haemoglobin; (*b*) decreased number of erythrocytes and shortened life span; (*c*) increased number of reticulocytes (young erythrocytes); and (*d*) increased number of basophilic stippled erythrocytes (manifestation of degenerated regeneration). Thus, a blood examination to detect these effects could be used as a measure of lead exposure. It should be noted that while the measurement of lead in urine and blood indicates lead exposure, the biochemical and haematological tests, though lacking in specificity, could be used to determine the duration of exposure and intensity of adverse effects.

Independently, none of the above tests can be regarded as diagnostic. However, two or more of them may be used together to assess exposure (past or present) and to determine the form of clinical poisoning (acute or chronic). Haematological tests are least specific, but may be useful and supportive. In sampling blood, great care should be taken to avoid lead contamination. The timing of blood and urine samples is not crucial. Nevertheless, it is preferable to take blood or urine samples more than three to four days after the last exposure.

Clinical effects

Lead may exert toxic effects on the gastrointestinal, haematopoietic, nervous (peripheral and central), and renal systems.

Effects on the gastrointestinal system

Intestinal colic (spasms of the small intestines) is the commonest clinical manifestation of developed lead poisoning. It is usually preceded, and almost invariably accompanied, by severe constipation. The pain is localized around or below the umbilicus. A sign of lead exposure (not related to colic) is a greyish pigmentation of the gums ("lead line").

Effects on the haematopoietic system

Lead inhibits the activity of the enzyme δ-aminolevulinate dehydratase (ALAD) in erythroblasts in the bone marrow and in the erythrocytes. This leads to increased concentrations of δ-ALA in the serum and urine. Clustered ribosomes are visible in the basophilic stippled cells as punctate basophilia even in the absence of anaemia. High levels of ALAD may have a neurotoxic action.

Effects on the nervous system

Cerebral involvement may vary with the age of the patient (children and young adults are particularly susceptible), the intensity of exposure, and additional exposure to other toxic substances (e.g., alcohol). The most serious manifestations of acute encephalopathy are of three types: convulsive, comatose, and delirious.

These effects of lead may not be completely reversible and the risk of permanent complications increases with repeated exposure. The most prominent abnormalities in chronic and subclinical encephalopathy include: slowness of performance; psychomotor disturbances; slight intelligence defects; and personality changes.

Alkyl compounds of lead cause a special form of encephalopathy (toxic psychosis) with insomnia or terrifying dreams in early cases, and different symptom complexes (delirious, manic, confused, schizophrenic) in severe cases.

Effects on the renal system

During the acute phase of lead poisoning, there is often functional renal involvement, but permanent renal damage is not certain. Later, the kidneys excrete less lead and a moderate degree of interstitial fibrosis may develop. A third phase (renal failure) has been postulated but has never been confirmed in adults. Lead may contribute to the renal disease of patients with gout; this and other reported effects are not considered to be conclusive.

Exposure–effect/relationship

According to present knowledge, blood lead concentrations of less than 400 μg/litre do not cause adverse neurological effects. Women are more likely to present impairment of erythropoiesis than men; in women the zinc protoporphyrin concentrations increase even at blood lead concentrations of about 300 µg/litre.

Prognosis

Chronic renal failure due to lead and acute lead encephalopathy may be fatal. Severe peripheral lead neuropathy may be irreversible, resulting in permanent paralysis.

Differential diagnosis

Acute intermittent porphyria and related abdominal and neuromuscular disorders may resemble acute lead poisoning. In both conditions the concentration of δ-ALA in urine is increased, but in porphyria there is no inhibition of ALAD. Lead colic, with its persistent constipation, is sometimes mistaken for an acute abdominal emergency.

Susceptibility

Women are more susceptible than men. In alcoholics there is a greater risk of nervous system damage than in non-alcoholics. Persons with nasal obstruction may also be at increased risk, since mouth breathing favours inhalation of larger dust particles. Malnutrition, haemoglobinopathies and enzymopathies, such as anaemias and glucose-6-phosphate dehydrogenase deficiency, and high lead body burden from previous occupational or non-occupational exposure also increase susceptibility.

Health examinations

Preplacement examination

The preplacement examination should include a medical history and a physical examination with special attention to haematopoietic, nervous, and renal systems. Blood haemoglobin should also be measured.

Periodic examination

In medical terms, the periodic examination is the same as the preplacement one. It is usually done annually. Besides examining the workers for the well known clinical signs and symptoms of lead exposure, laboratory tests that measure excessive lead absorption and those that confirm the toxic action of lead should be carried out. The criteria for excessive lead absorption can be arbitrarily indicated as follows:

lead in blood	> 2.896 µmol/litre (600 µg/litre)
protoporphyrin in erythrocytes	> 1.779 µmol/litre (1000 µg/litre) erythrocytes
zinc protoporphyrin in erythrocytes	> 0.54 mmol/mol haemoglobin
δ-aminolevulinic acid in urine	> 152.52 µmol/litre (20 mg/litre)
coproporphyrin in urine	> 0.459 mmol/litre (300 mg/litre)

Screening tests

The concentrations of lead in blood and protoporphyrin in erythrocytes (or coproporphyrin or δ-aminolevulinic acid in urine, depending upon the laboratory) should be measured at 3–6-month intervals. The frequency of such screening tests depends upon the level of potential exposure and the results of previous health examinations and screening tests.

Case management

Workers with excessive lead absorption should be removed from further exposure until the measurements indicated under *Periodic examination* fall below the critical values.

For therapy of lead poisoning, chelating agents such as calcium disodium ethylenediaminotetraacetate ($CaNa_2EDTA$) or penicillamine are used. Oral $CaNa_2EDTA$ should never be used for prophylaxis.

Control measures

Strict attention should be paid to any source of lead dust or fumes and technical control measures should be applied wherever necessary. Industrial and personal hygiene are of great importance. Food and drink must not be brought into the workrooms, and smoking at work must not be allowed.

Exposure limits for lead in air vary in different countries from $0.001 \, mg/m^3$ to $0.15 \, mg/m^3$. A WHO Study Group[1] has recommended a health-based occupational exposure limit for lead in blood of 400 µg/litre for males and females over the reproductive age and 300 µg/litre for females in reproductive age. For δ-aminolevulinic acid in urine, no increase over the laboratory's "normal" upper limit (e.g., mean + 2 SD) should occur. In the case of zinc protoporphyrin in urine, the normal level may be raised by up to 50%. With regard to lead in air, a range of 30–60 µg/m³ was recommended.

---

[1] WHO Technical Report Series, No. 647, 1980.

CHAPTER 15

Diseases caused by fluorine and its toxic compounds

Properties of the causal agents

Elemental fluorine is a yellow, highly reactive gas. The fluorine compounds of concern in industry are derived from fluorspar (CaF_2) and cryolite (sodium aluminium fluoride, Na_3AlF_6).

Occurrence and uses

Fluorine and its compounds as encountered in industry are largely derived from phosphate rock processing, which yields fluosilicic acid. Apart from the comparatively small amounts of gaseous fluorine, the element is largely found, in industry as in nature, in chemically combined form (the fluorides). Fluorides are mainly used in steel fluxing, the manufacture of bricks, tiles, pottery, cement, glass, enamel, and fibreglass, and in aluminium smelting. Fluorine and hydrogen fluoride are used in the synthesis of fluorocarbons, gasoline production (as an alkylating catalyst), metal casting operations and welding, rocket fuel systems, metalplating, and surface heating operations.

Occupations involving exposure to fluorides

Workers in phosphate fertilizer manufacture, open hearth and basic oxygen furnaces in steel plants, and aluminium reduction cell room operations and cryolite plant or fluorspar miners are at greatest risk. Others who may also be exposed include cement, porcelain enamel, magnesium foundry, and certain electroplating workers.

Mechanism of action

Absorption

The gaseous (F, HF) as well as particulate forms are readily absorbed through the lung at the alveolar level. Particulates deposited above this level are raised by the mucociliary escalator mechanism, swallowed, and ultimately absorbed in large part in the gastrointestinal tract.

Distribution

Approximately 25% of blood fluoride is in the plasma, the remainder being in or on erythrocytes. The plasma contains fluoride both in the ionic form (20% of total blood fluorine) and as bound, nonexchangeable fluoride. Essentially, all organs and tissues contain fluoride (in intracellular water), but the highest concentrations of fluoride (99% of total fluorine body burden) are found in the bones as fluorapatite.

Excretion

The principal route of excretion is via the urine. Renal clearance is rapid, with approximately 60% of the absorbed amount being excreted within 24 hours of exposure. About 10% of the absorbed amount appears in faeces, and negligible amounts are found in sweat, hair, breast milk, and saliva.

Assessment of exposure

Environmental assessment

The most precise measure of occupational exposure to most fluorides is air sampling in the breathing zone, preferably by personal sampling pumps that draw air through a sodium formate-treated filter. In the case of hydrogen fluoride, a direct reading of its air concentration may be made by appropriate detector tubes.

Biological assessment

The most practical indicator of fluorine body burden is the concentration of fluorides in the urine, which can be accurately and quickly measured with ion-specific electrodes. Information on the routine use of serum fluoride determinations is at present insufficient.

Fluorine in urine. Human urinary fluoride concentrations depend upon—and, in fact are, numerically, quite close to—the drinking-water concentrations. When drinking-water contains little fluoride, urinary concentrations are in the range of 0.2–0.5 mg/litre. Where water contains 1 mg fluoride/litre, urine concentrations range from 0.5 mg/litre to 1.5 mg/litre. Tea drinking may increase urinary fluoride concentration by 50–100%. People living in areas with highly fluoridated waters (e.g., up to 8–9 mg fluoride/litre) show comparable concentrations in urine.

Because fluoride rapidly appears in the urine following the commencement of exposure, the urinary concentration obtained at the end of a workshift approximately represents fluoride exposure during the workshift. However, the most accurate measure of exposure during a workshift is the concentration obtained at the end of the workshift on the third to fifth day of the work week. Exposures greater than 2.5–3 mg/m^3 (time-weighted average) will yield urinary fluoride concentrations at the end of the workshift in excess of 8 mg/litre.

In order to assess the body burden of fluorine, (which is mainly the amount of fluoride in the bones), at least two days' removal from exposure is essential before urine sampling.

Clinical effects

The effects of occupational exposure to fluorides take many years to become manifest. According to historical literature, even after exposure to extreme concentrations of fluoride in air (ranging from 20 mg/m^3 to 9 g/m^3), it took approximately 10 years for the earliest detectable bone changes to occur.

Acute poisoning

Acute poisoning may occur after exposure to high concentrations in air of fluorine and hydrogen fluoride. In such cases, there is immediate irritation of the exposed tissues, including the eyes and the respiratory tract. However, acute poisoning rarely occurs in occupational settings because both fluorine and hydrogen fluoride are quickly detected by their smell and workers are likely to hold their breath and move away from the contaminated area.

Chronic poisoning

The most significant consequence of excessive fluoride exposure is the damage to the skeletal system and associated tissues. The first stage of osteofluorosis consists of an increase in the density of pelvic and vertebral bones, with coarseness and blurring of bone trabeculae. The evaluation of such changes is very difficult since there are no specific symptoms or metabolic or physical consequences in the first stage. Furthermore, expertise in this area is limited. Only those with many years' experience of dealing with cases of fluorosis can be expected to make an accurate diagnosis at this stage.

After some years, the second stage ensues. At this stage there is increased density and blurring of contours of the pelvic and vertebral bones, ribs, and extremities. Calcification of the sacrotuberous and sacrosciatic ligaments is uniquely seen in osteofluorosis. However, symptoms or functional alterations related to the changes in the bones are nonspecific and inconsistent.

At the third stage crippling fluorosis occurs. There is greatly increased bone density with blurring and irregularity of bone contours throughout the body, especially in cancellous bone. There is considerable calcification of ligaments, especially those of the neck and vertebral column. In contrast to the first two stages, this rare complication can produce marked restriction of locomotion.

It has been suggested that fluoride exposure has damaging consequences on the respiratory system. However, more data are needed to clarify the question of the specific role of fluoride.

Exposure–effect relationship

A concentration of airborne fluorine of $5 \, mg/m^3$ may cause eye and respiratory tract irritation in some persons. Evidence from several sources indicates that urinary fluoride concentrations not exceeding 5 mg/litre in pre-workshift samples taken after two days of removal from exposure are not associated with detectable osteosclerosis, and that such changes are unlikely even at urinary concentrations of up to 8 mg/litre. At air concentrations of fluoride persistently exceeding $2.5 \, mg/m^3$ and post-workshift urinary concentrations equal to or exceeding 9 mg/litre, first-stage osteofluorosis can be expected in some workers after many years' exposure, usually greater than 15–20 years. A fluorine content of bones of 4000–6000 mg/kg (dry, fat-free) is consistent with first-stage osteofluorosis. When removed from exposure, persons with first-stage osteofluorosis show urinary concentrations of 5–6 mg of fluoride per litre or greater and these levels persist for long periods.

Prognosis

Even if osteofluorosis progresses to stage two, there is usually little evidence of physical, functional, or metabolic changes in the bones. However, with a reasonable degree of surveillance, it is possible to prevent the progression of the disease to such an extent.

Differential diagnosis

The increase in the density of the pelvic and vertebral bones in osteofluorosis differs from sclerosing osteitis, a condition that occurs mainly in children and is accompanied by severe anaemia and skull changes. Such changes are never seen in osteofluorosis.

Susceptibility

Except for individuals whose renal function is compromised, there is no particular group of persons at special risk. Transplacental transfer of fluoride is apparently not affected.

Health examinations

The measurement of urinary fluoride concentrations on a periodic basis is the most important method for the early detection and prevention of osteofluorosis. Precipitous intervention is rarely useful or indicated.

Preplacement examination

The preplacement examination should include a medical history and a physical examination, with special attention to musculoskeletal, pulmonary, and urinary systems. A baseline radiograph of the pelvis should be taken and retained. Urinary fluoride concentration should be determined.

Periodic examination

In medical terms, the periodic examination is the same as the preplacement one. It is usually done annually. At this examination, the urinary fluoride concentrations are measured after at least 48-hours' removal from exposure. Urine samples with a relative density of less than 1.005 should be discarded. If the concentration is around 5 mg/litre, the test should be repeated. If the fluoride concentration remains persistently high, workplace hygiene and ventilation status and dietary and work habits should be investigated and appropriate control measures introduced. In adequately controlled workplaces, urine fluoride concentrations are mostly in the range of 1.5–3 mg/litre. If persistent urinary fluoride concentrations above 5 mg/litre occur, renal function should be investigated and a pelvic X-ray should be taken, care being exercised to protect the gonads.

Screening tests

Every six months after the third to fifth day of the working week, a urine sample should be taken (for fluoride analysis) after showering. If the fluoride concentration is found to be around 8 mg/litre the test should be repeated. If the fluoride concentrations in urine remain persistently high, work practices and hygienic conditions should be reviewed and appropriate measures taken to reduce exposure.

If in a group of workers the pre-workshift urinary fluoride values exceed a geometric mean of 5 mg/litre, or if the geometric mean concentration after the workshift exceeds 7 mg/litre, the working conditions of the group should be reviewed.

Case management

If in an individual the urinary fluoride concentrations taken after an exposure-free period of 48 hours remain consistently above 5 mg/litre for several years (8–10 years) his removal from exposure should be considered. At stage one of osteofluorosis the removal of patients from work-related exposure will prevent further health impairment. The absence of exposure may permit very slow clearance of fluoride from the bones, so long as renal function is intact.

Control measures

Adequate technical controls and scrupulous management of work hygiene are extremely important. The enclosure of fume- and dust-producing operations is usually quite effective. Practices to minimize dust dispersion in work areas, such as vacuum sweeping, are necessary. Facilities for the maintenance of good personal hygiene should be provided. Food should be stored in uncontaminated areas and washing of hands before eating should be insisted upon. Lunchrooms should have positive-pressure ventilation, and eating and smoking should be prohibited in work areas. Tobacco and foodstuffs should not be carried in fluoride-contaminated clothing and cigarettes be carried only in closed cases.

Exposure limits for fluorine in different countries are between 0.05 mg/m³ and 2 mg/m³; the limits for fluorides (as fluorine) range from 1 mg/m³ to 2.5 mg/m³.

CHAPTER 16

Diseases caused by carbon disulfide

Properties of the causal agent

Pure carbon disulfide (CS_2) is a colourless, highly refractive liquid of sweetish aromatic odour. Commercial and reagent grade CS_2 is a yellowish liquid with a foul smell. It is volatile and flammable, and its vapours are explosive.

Occurrence and uses

Carbon disulfide may be present in minute quantities in coal tar and crude petroleum. It is commercially produced by heating charcoal with vapourized sulfur and also by reacting sulfur with petroleum hydrocarbons. Its main use is in the viscose rayon industry as a solvent of alkaline cellulose. It is also used as a solvent in laboratories, and various industrial processes, and in the production of flotation agents and herbicides.

Occupations involving risk of exposure to carbon disulfide

Occupational exposure is mainly confined to the viscose industry, where carbon disulfide vapours are released concomitantly with hydrogen sulfide (H_2S).

Mechanism of action

Absorption

CS_2 is absorbed mainly as vapour by inhalation. An equilibrium between inhaled and exhaled carbon disulfide is reached in 1–2 h, with about 40–50 % of the inhaled vapours being retained. Skin absorption is possible from direct contact with liquid carbon disulfide.

Biotransformation

Of the absorbed carbon disulfide 70–90 % undergoes biotransformation into dithiocarbamic acids and isothiocyanates.

Excretion

Less than 1 % of the absorbed amount is excreted unchanged in the urine; 70–90 % is metabolized (as noted above) and excreted in the urine. The rest is eliminated by exhalation and in saliva and sweat.

Assessment of exposure

Environmental assessment

The methods for the measurement of carbon disulfide concentrations in the workroom air include: (*a*) gas-detection tubes; (*b*) photometric analysis of air samples absorbed in liquid sorbents; (*c*) analysis of air samples adsorbed on activated charcoal by gas–liquid chromatography; and (*d*) gas analysers that give continuous direct readings.

For regular monitoring of exposure, time-weighted average air concentrations should be measured, either by area sampling in the breathing zone or, preferably, by personal sampling.

Biological assessment

At exposure levels higher than 50 mg of CS_2/m^3 of air, the iodine–azide test reflects exposure to carbon disulfide quantitatively. This test is based on the fact that the metabolites of carbon disulfide excreted in the urine catalyse the reaction between iodine and sodium azide. One urine sample should be collected at the end of the working day and another before the workshift on the following day. At exposure levels lower than 50 mg/m^3, the iodine–azide test yields negative results.

Clinical effects

Carbon disulfide is primarily a neurotoxic poison. Repeated exposure to high concentrations may cause damage to many body systems. Long-term exposures to low concentrations may result in mental, neurological, cardiovascular, gastrointestinal, metabolic, endocrinological, and other effects.

Acute poisoning

Exposure to about 10 g/m^3 may cause coma or even death. Repeated exposure to CS_2 concentrations of 3–5 g/m^3 may result in different psychiatric and neurological signs and symptoms, including extreme irritability, hallucinations, manic delirium, paranoia, and other disturbances.

Chronic poisoning

Long-term exposure over many years may produce a syndrome of chronic poisoning manifested by a variety of signs and symptoms arising from the manifold adverse effects on different organs and systems. Chronic encephalopathy is associated with psychological and behavioural changes. As poisoning progresses, neurological signs predominate. Both pyramidal and extrapyramidal syndromes develop, as well as disturbances in autonomic nervous centres and signs of more diffuse cortical involvement. Vascular changes are probably responsible for much of the central nervous system pathology. Symmetrical polyneuropathy affects mainly the sensory nerves of the lower extremities.

Under present working conditions, subjective symptoms (pains, paraesthesiae, cramps in the lower limbs, disturbances of memory and emotional changes) and neurophysiological changes (reduced nerve conduction velocity and electromyographic signs of neurogenic lesions) are mostly seen.

Vascular changes due to carbon disulfide exposure are similar to those of atherosclerosis in older age groups. Long-term exposure to carbon disulfide promotes coronary heart disease, even under circumstances in which clinical poisoning is uncommon. An increased frequency of retinal microaneurysms has been reported.

Gastrointestinal symptoms, including dyspepsia, gastritis, and ulcerative changes have been noted in workers exposed to high concentrations of carbon disulfide.

Effects on the endocrine system include: (a) reduction in the activity of the adrenal gland as a result of reduced secretion of corticotropin; (b) impairment of spermatogenesis, and (c) disturbance of the hormonal balance in women, evidenced by menstrual irregularities, spontaneous abortions, and premature deliveries. Thyroid function may also be affected.

In recent years, owing to improved industrial hygiene, the pattern of CS_2 intoxications described in the literature has changed from heavy psychiatric and neurological symptomatology to latent subtle alterations detectable only by means of sophisticated tests.

Delayed effects

There are no reports of any carcinogenic, mutagenic, or teratogenic effects of carbon disulfide.

Exposure–effect relationship

Air concentrations of around 60–90 mg/m³ may produce psychological effects. An excess of vascular effects (involving the brain and heart) has been reported in workers subjected to long-term exposure to concentrations averaging 30–125 mg/m³. Some studies indicate that concentrations below about 60 mg/m³, and perhaps even below 10 mg/m³, may cause some physiological disturbances.

Prognosis

While the prognosis of acute poisoning is favourable, that of the effects of chronic exposure depends upon the organs and systems involved and on the severity of the effects. Behavioural, neurological, and vascular changes may last for several years even after the cessation of exposure, and in some cases they may be permanent.

Differential diagnosis

Acute poisoning

Other illnesses and conditions that result in a confused mental state or coma (central nervous system affections, diabetes, etc.) should be excluded. High-level exposure to carbon disulfide in the workroom air should be proved by the iodine–azide test.

Chronic poisoning

Other mental and neurological disorders should be excluded. It is not possible to differentiate between cardiovascular disorders caused by CS_2 and those due to other causes.

Because there is no pathognomonic sign of chronic CS_2 poisoning, (i.e., all changes are nonspecific), the diagnosis of the effects of CS_2 exposure depends on the ascertainment of exposure (by environmental and biological monitoring), exclusion of other diseases, and the demonstration of symptoms and signs of intoxication and their combinations.

Susceptibility

Persons at greatest risk include: young people; pregnant women; persons with mental illness; and persons suffering from disturbances of the autonomic nervous system, diseases of the central and peripheral nervous systems, gastritis, peptic ulcers and other chronic gastrointestinal conditions, metabolic diseases, cardiovascular diseases, or from pulmonary or other conditions that prevent the use of respirators. Also at risk are subjects showing a positive iodine–azide test in pre-workshift urine samples.

Health examinations

Preplacement examination

The preplacement examination should include a medical history and a physical examination, with special attention to the nervous and cardiovascular systems. In addition, depending on the level of exposure and the age and health of the subject, an electrocardiogram may be taken (preferably in conjunction with an exercise test), the serum high-density lipoprotein cholesterol may be determined, and opthalmoscopy (to detect possible retinopathy) may be performed.

Periodic examination

In medical terms, the periodic examination is the same as the preplacement one. It should be performed once or twice a year. Additional examinations include ocular fundus photography, examination of the blood–lipid pattern (in high exposure), behavioural testing, electromyography electroencephalography, measurement of nerve conduction velocity, and colour discrimination testing.

Screening test

Depending on level of exposure, the iodine–azide test should be carried out several times a year, both immediately after the workshift and the following morning before starting work.

Case management

Workers suffering from chronic poisoning or from adverse effects of repeated accidental exposures must be removed from exposure permanently. There is no specific treatment.

Control measures

Exposure should be limited by enclosing processes involving carbon disulfide as well as by general and local exhaust ventilation. Continuous supervision with a view to ensuring sound work practice, and the use of personal protection devices against respiratory and skin absorption is also essential.

Exposure limits for carbon disulfide in air in different countries vary from 1 mg/m^3 to 60 mg/m^3. In 1981, a WHO Study Group[1] recommended that the short-term exposure limit (15 min) should not exceed 60 mg/m^3 during the working day, with the time-weighted average being maintained at 10 mg/m^3 for male workers and 3 mg/m^3 (tentative) for female workers of reproductive age.

---

[1] WHO Technical Report Series, No. 664, 1981.

CHAPTER 17

Diseases caused by toxic halogen derivatives of aliphatic and aromatic hydrocarbons

Introduction

Aliphatic halogenated hydrocarbons are compounds of carbon, hydrogen, and halogens (chlorine, bromine, fluorine). They may be saturated or unsaturated carbon chains in which one or more hydrogen atoms have been replaced by one or more halogens. They are mainly colourless, volatile liquids, and are excellent solvents of organic compounds. However, most of the fluorinated compounds (fluorocarbons) are colourless, nonflammable gases. The aliphatic halogenated hydrocarbons decompose easily on exposure to heat or open flame, releasing some highly irritant compounds such as phosgene and hydrofluoric acid. They are widely used as solvents in degreasing, dewaxing, dry-cleaning, and extraction processes. They are also used as aerosol propellants, refrigerants, fumigants, insecticides, fire extinguishers, and as chemical intermediates in organic synthesis. The fluorocarbons are used as refrigerants, aerosol propellants, polymer intermediates, and anaesthetics.

Aromatic halogenated hydrocarbons are derived from benzene, its homologues, and other aromatic compounds by the replacement of one or more hydrogen atoms by halogens. Chlorinated benzenes are liquids, whereas the physical states of chlorinated diphenyls and their derivatives and chlorinated naphthalenes vary from liquids to waxy solids, depending on the degree of chlorination.

Aromatic halogenated hydrocarbons are used as chemical intermediates in the production of dyes, pharmaceuticals, pesticides, plastics, etc. Chlorinated biphenyls and naphthalenes, owing to their stability, thermoplasticity, and non-flammability, are used as electrical insulators (in capacitors and cables) and as additives in extreme-pressure lubricants.

Both these groups of compounds include a large number of chemicals of industrial importance and it is not possible to discuss all of them here. However, the most important ones are summarized in Table 2, which also provides basic information about their uses and properties. A number of selected compounds are considered in the sections below.

102

Table 2. Uses and toxic properties of some industrially important aliphatic and aromatic halogenated hydrocarbons

Substance	Main uses	Target organ or tissue	Degree of toxicity[a]	
			Acute	Chronic
Methyl chloride (CH_3Cl)	Chemical syntheses (methylation), refrigerant, special extraction agent	CNS[b] liver	+++ +	+++
Methylene chloride (CH_2Cl_2)	Solvent (oils, fats, waxes, cellulose acetate), degreaser, paint remover	CNS	+	+
Chloroform ($CHCl_3$)	Solvent (lacquers), extraction agent	CNS liver	+++ ++	+ +
Carbon tetrachloride (CCl_4) (see also page 105)	Chemical syntheses, fire extinguishers (for use as a solvent should be replaced by less toxic substance)	CNS liver kidneys	++ +++ +++	+ +++ ++
Ethyl chloride (CH_3CH_2Cl)	Chemical syntheses, local anaesthetic (freezing)	CNS	++	Not known
1,2-dichloroethane ($ClCH_2CH_2Cl$)	Chemical syntheses, solvent (resins, rubber, bitumen, paints), degreaser, extraction agent for oils etc.	CNS liver kidney	++	+ +
1,1,1-trichloroethane (CH_3CCl_3)	Degreasing agent in metal cleaning and dry-cleaning; good substitute for carbon tetrachloride	CNS	+++	++
1,1,2-trichloroethane ($CH_2ClCHCl_2$)	Solvent (should be replaced by less toxic substances)	Same as carbon tetrachloride		
tetrachloroethane ($CHCl_2CHCl_2$)	Solvent (should be replaced by less toxic substances)	Same as carbon tetrachloride		

Table 2. (Contd.)

Substance	Main uses	Target organ or tissue	Degree of toxicity[a]	
			Acute	Chronic
trichloroethylene (ClCH=CCl$_2$) (see also page 108)	Degreaser, dry-cleaning and extraction agent, chemical syntheses	CNS	+++	+++
tetrachloroethylene (Cl$_2$C=CCl$_2$)	Degreaser, dry-cleaning and extraction agent, chemical syntheses	CNS	+++	+
vinyl chloride (CH$_2$=CHCl) (see also page 118)	Intermediate in the manufacture of poly-vinylchloride	CNS liver, bones	+	+++ +++
methyl bromide (CH$_3$Br)	Insect fumigant (grain), chemical syntheses	CNS	+++	+++
ethyl bromide (CH$_3$CH$_2$Br)	Chemical syntheses, special extraction agent	CNS	++	Not known
1,2-dibromoethane (BrCH$_2$CH$_2$Br)	Insect fumigant (soil), fire extinguisher, solvent (celluloid, fats, oils, waxes)	CNS liver kidneys	++ ++ +	+ ++ +
chlorobenzene (C$_6$H$_5$Cl)	Chemical syntheses, solvent	CNS liver mucous membranes	++ ++ +	Not known
dichlorobenzene (C$_6$H$_4$Cl$_2$)	Chemical syntheses, insecticide	CNS liver mucous membranes	+++ ++ ++	++ ++

[a] + = mildly toxic; ++ = moderately toxic; and +++ = highly toxic.
[b] Central nervous system.

CARBON TETRACHLORIDE

Properties of the causal agent

Carbon tetrachloride, (CCl_4) is a colourless, volatile liquid with a moderately strong ethereal odour. It boils at 76.8 °C but is not flammable.

Occurrence and uses

CCl_4 is produced by reacting carbon disulfide with chlorine in the presence of a catalyst or by the chlorination of methane. It is used as a substrate in the production of fluorocarbons. In fumigant mixtures, it is used as an insecticide and to suppress the flammability of more flammable fumigants. In recent years, its use as a solvent for oils, fats, lacquers, varnishes, and resins, has been regulated in various countries.

Occupations involving risk of exposure to carbon tetrachloride

Chemists, degreasers, grain fumigators, ink-makers, insecticide makers, and refrigerant makers are at greatest risk of exposure.

Mechanism of action

Absorption

Carbon tetrachloride is mainly absorbed through the lungs as vapour. Although absorption through intact skin is apparently slight, repeated contact with the skin should nevertheless be avoided.

Biotransformation

Carbon tetrachloride is metabolized in the liver to form a free radical ($\cdot CCl_3$), which causes cell damage through lipid peroxidation. Small amounts of carbon tetrachloride are metabolized to carbon dioxide and urea.

Elimination

About half the absorbed carbon tetrachloride is eliminated unchanged in the expired air (small amounts (4%) as CO_2) and the remainder is excreted in the urine and faeces, largely as metabolites.

Assessment of exposure

Environmental assessment

Exposure is assessed by analysing samples of workroom air in the breathing zone, preferably by a personal sampler. Samplers for CCl_4 consist of charcoal tubes that adsorb vapours from the air, subsequent analysis being done by gas chromatography. Detector tubes are also available for screening.

Biological assessment

At the present time, none of the metabolites of CCl_4 in blood or urine appears to be of value in monitoring exposure. Carbon tetrachloride in expired air may be useful in the diagnosis of acute exposure and also, possibly, in assessing the magnitude of exposure.

Clinical effects

Carbon tetrachloride causes central nervous system depression and severe damage to the liver and kidneys. In animals, it has produced liver tumours. Prolonged or repeated skin contact with the liquid may cause dermatitis.

Acute poisoning

Exposure to high concentrations results in symptoms of central nervous system depression, including dizziness, vertigo, lack of coordination, and mental confusion. Abdominal pain, nausea, vomiting, and diarrhoea are frequent. In animals, the primary damage from intoxication is to the liver, but in humans the majority of fatalities have been the result of renal injury with secondary cardiac failure. Human fatalities from acute renal damage have occurred after exposure for 30 minutes to 1 hour to concentrations of 6.5–13 g/m³; sudden deaths may have been caused occasionally by ventricular fibrillation. Liver damage results from the necrosis of the hepatic cells with fatty infiltration. In kidney damage, there is fatty degeneration and necrosis of the epithelium of renal tubules.

Within a few days of acute exposure, jaundice may appear and liver injury may progress to toxic necrosis. At the same time, acute nephritis may occur, with albumin, red and white blood cells, and casts appearing in the urine. There may be oliguria, anuria, and increased nitrogen retention, resulting in uraemia.

Chronic poisoning

Injury to the liver and kidneys can occur from a single acute exposure, but it is more frequently the result of repeated exposures.

Chronic exposure causes various vision abnormalities, such as reduced visual field. There is a synergistic effect from excessive alcohol intake and exposure to carbon tetrachloride. In many cases of poisoning, especially those involving severe liver and kidney damage, alcohol has been a concomitant factor.

Delayed effects

The International Agency for Research on Cancer recommends that carbon tetrachloride should be regarded as carcinogenic to humans. In rats and mice it produces liver tumours after administration by many routes.

Exposure–effect relationship

There are several reports of adverse effects (nausea, vomiting, dizziness, drowsiness, and headache) in workers repeatedly exposed to workroom air concentrations of CCl_4 between $160 \, mg/m^3$ and $200 \, mg/m^3$. A reduction in the visual field occurred in workers repeatedly exposed to concentrations between $40 \, mg/m^3$ and $65 \, mg/m^3$.

Prognosis

The prognosis of liver and kidney damage is favourable if the workers are removed from further exposure early enough.

Differential diagnosis

Acute poisoning

Other causes of mental confusion, particularly affections of the central nervous and cardiovascular systems (whether metabolic or toxic in origin) should be excluded. Evidence of high-level exposure (work history, smell of carbon tetrachloride in breath, high concentration of carbon tetrachloride in breath or blood) must be present.

Chronic poisoning

Other causes of diffuse liver diseases (such as viral hepatitis and alcoholic liver disease) and other causes of kidney disease (such as other toxic nephroses, glomerulonephritis, and systemic diseases affecting the glomerulus and renal haemodynamics) should be excluded.

Susceptibility

Persons suffering from liver and kidney disease are believed to be more susceptible than others.

Health examinations

Preplacement examination

The preplacement health examination should include a medical history, a physical examination, liver function tests, renal function tests, and urinalysis.

Periodic examination

A medical examination should be carried out annually, with emphasis on the liver, kidneys, and skin. Liver function tests, renal function tests, and urinalysis should also be done.

Case management

In acute poisoning or skin and eye contamination, remove the worker from exposure, wash the affected skin areas, and irrigate the eyes with water. It may be necessary to treat for shock. In cases of oliguria and anuria, give fluids and electrolytes. Dialysis should be considered in severe cases. Treat central nervous system depression or liver disease symptomatically.

Control measures

Exposure to carbon tetrachloride should be kept as low as possible by employing technical control procedures and by personal protection devices. Exposure limits for carbon tetrachloride in different countries range from $1 \, \text{mg/m}^3$ to $65 \, \text{mg/m}^3$.

TRICHLOROETHYLENE

Properties of the causal agent

Trichloroethylene $ClCH = CCl_2$ is a clear colourless liquid with a typical sweet odour. It is a very good organic solvent. Technical grade trichloroethylene used for degreasing purposes often contains several compounds as additives (e.g., 1,2-epoxybutane, epichlorohydrin).

Occurrence and uses

Trichloroethylene is produced by treating trichloroethane with lime or alkali in the presence of water. It is used in degreasing metal parts, dry-cleaning of clothes, extracting oils and fats, and as a thinner for paints, lacquers, varnishes, and tar and as a solvent for rubber.

Occupations involving exposure to trichloroethylene

Chemists engaged in the production and use of trichloroethylene, degreasers, dry cleaners, fat processors, etc. are at greatest risk of exposure.

Mechanism of action

Absorption

Trichloroethylene is absorbed mainly as vapour through the lungs. A limited amount may also be absorbed through intact skin upon direct contact with the liquid. About 60% of the absorbed amount is retained.

Biotransformation

About 70–90% of the absorbed amount is metabolized, mainly to trichloroethanol and trichloroacetic acid.

Excretion

About 10–20% of the absorbed amount is exhaled unchanged. Its metabolites are excreted in the urine. Whereas the majority of the trichloroethanol is eliminated within the first 24 hours after exposure, the elimination of most of the trichloroacetic acid takes place over 2–3 days, because the latter is bound to proteins. In individuals with prolonged continuous exposure, the ratio of the concentration of trichloroethanol to that of trichloroacetic acid in the urine is about 2:1.

Assessment of exposure

Environmental assessment

Detector tubes may be used for the determination of air concentration in cases of emergency, before entering confined spaces, or for screening purposes. For quantitative measurements of air concentration, direct-reading instruments, infrared spectrophotometry, and gas chromatography may be used. Adsorption of trichloroethylene vapour on charcoal-filled tubes is a convenient method for personal sampling.

Biological assessment

The determination of trichloroethylene metabolites in the urine by spectrophotometry (Fujiwara reaction) or by gas chromatography is the method of choice. Owing to individual variability valid results are obtainable only on a group basis. While the urinary concentration of trichloroethanol (which is excreted rapidly) chiefly reflects the recent exposure level, that of trichloroacetic acid indicates the cumulative exposure over several days. Therefore, post-workshift urine samples obtained after 3–4 successive days of work should be used for the assessment of exposure. The relationship between trichloroethylene in air (mg/m^3) and its metabolites in urine (mole per mole of creatinine with figures in mg per g of creatinine in parentheses) are as follows:

Trichloroethylene in air	Trichloroethanol	Trichloroacetic acid	Total trichloroethylene metabolites
270 mg/m^3	0.095–0.15 mol/mol (125–200 mg/g)	0.052–0.087 mol/mol (75–125 mg/g)	(200–300 mg/g)
540 mg/m^3	0.19–0.3 mol/mol (250–400 mg/g)	0.1–0.17 mol/mol (150–250 mg/g)	(400–600 mg/g)

Clinical effects

Acute poisoning

Exposure to high concentrations of trichloroethylene results in central nervous system depression (dizziness, vertigo, lack of coordination, confusion, coma). Long-term contact of unconscious patients with liquid trichloroethylene may cause blistering of the skin. Chemical pneumonitis and some degree of liver and kidney damage are also possible.

Chronic poisoning

The nervous system is the main target and psychosomatic complaints are the main symptoms (fatigue, sleep disorders, changes of mood, impairment of memory, intolerance of alcohol, etc.). These symptoms may be accompanied by dispersed minor neurological signs (mainly affecting the brain-stem structures and autonomic nervous system), and psychological deterioration. Some biochemical changes related to liver function impairment (e.g., mildly elevated blood concentrations of aminotransferases) are also possible, but serious liver disease has not been observed. Dermatitis may develop owing to the defatting effect of liquid trichloroethylene.

Delayed effects

Animal experiments indicate that technical grade trichloroethylene may be carcinogenic. In this regard, the role of additives has been suspected. Although an increase in cancer incidence has not been found in workers exposed to trichloroethylene, the risk cannot be ruled out.

Exposure–effect relationship

In short-term exposure, no adverse effects on neuropsychological functions have been observed at air concentrations ranging between 510 mg/m^3 and 540 mg/m^3. In long-term exposure, some adverse effects on the nervous system have been observed at exposures resulting in average urinary concentrations of trichloroacetic acid of above 0.306 mmol/litre (50 mg/litre). The corresponding concentration of trichloroethylene in air would be above 135 mg/m^3.

Prognosis

In acute poisoning by inhalation, most symptoms disappear promptly with the breathing of uncontaminated air and elimination of the absorbed trichloroethylene and its metabolites. The neurological or psychological disturbances may last longer. The prognosis of chronic poisoning is favourable after removal of the worker from further exposure.

Differential diagnosis

Acute poisoning

Exclude other causes of disturbed consciousness (neurological and metabolic disorders such as diabetes). The diagnosis should be based on evidence of high-level exposure (work history, smell of trichloroethylene in breath, metabolites in urine).

Chronic poisoning

Other neurological affections should be excluded. Evidence of high-level occupational exposure (work history, high concentrations of trichloroethylene in air and urine) is important for diagnosis.

Susceptibility

Pre-existing neurological and psychiatric diseases possibly indicate higher sensitivity.

Health examinations

Preplacement examination

The preplacement health examination should include a medical history and a physical examination, with special attention to the nervous system, liver, and skin.

Periodic examination

In medical terms, the periodic examination is the same as the preplacement one. Under usual working conditions this examination rarely needs to be repeated more frequently than once a year.

Case management

In acute poisoning, first immediately remove the individual from further exposure. Then remove clothes that may have become contaminated and wash all the affected skin areas with soap and water. Give treatment according to the individual's symptoms. If necessary, give artificial respiration.

In chronic poisoning, remove the patient from further exposure until he is fully recovered.

Control measures

Owing to the possible carcinogenicity of tricholoroethylene, exposure to it should be kept as low as possible by appropriate technical control measures.

Exposure limits for trichloroethylene in different countries range from 10 mg/m^3 to 535 mg/m^3. A WHO Study Group[1] recommended that during a working day, the short-term (15-min) peak concentrations should not exceed 1000 mg/m^3, and a time-weighted average of 135 mg/m^3 should be maintained.

HEXACHLORONAPHTHALENE

Properties of the causal agent

Hexachloronaphthalene ($C_{10}H_2Cl_6$) is a waxy white solid.

---

[1] WHO Technical Report Series, No. 664, 1981.

Uses

Hexachloronaphthalene is used in the production of electrical capacitors, the insulation of electric cables and wires, and the manufacture of storage batteries. It is also used as an additive in extreme-pressure lubricants and as a coating in foundry use. Industrial exposure to individual chlorinated naphthalenes is rare and usually occurs from mixtures of two or more species. Hexachloronaphthalene is often mixed with pentachloronaphthalene.

Occupations involving risk of exposure to hexachloronaphthalene

Cable coaters, capacitor impregnators, electrical workers, petrochemical workers, and rubber workers are at greatest risk.

Mechanism of action

Absorption

Hexachloronaphthalene enters the body by inhalation in the form of fumes from hot liquid, and absorption takes place mainly through the lungs. Absorption through intact skin may also occur upon direct contact with liquid hexachloronaphthalene.

Biotransformation

The main final metabolites are the hydroxylated derivatives and the hydroxylated dechlorinated derivatives.

Elimination

Hexachloronapthalene is excreted in the urine and faeces.

Assessment of exposure

Environmental assessment

The method of choice is air sampling in the breathing zone (preferably by personal sampling) using samplers with cellulose membrane filters, followed by gas chromatographic analysis.

Biological assessment

There are no special tests in common use.

Clinical effects

Acute poisoning

Acute poisoning by hexachloronaphthalene is not documented in the literature.

Chronic poisoning

Chronic exposure causes chloracne, which appears as simple erythematous eruptions with pustules, papules, and comedones. Cysts may develop owing to plugging of the sebaceous gland orifices. Fumes are the most potent chloracnegens, solutions are less so, and the solid rarely cause acne.

Chloracne is usually persistent and affects the face, ears, neck, shoulders, arms, chest, and abdomen (especially around the umbilicus and on the scrotum). The skin is frequently dry with intense pruritis, noninflammatory comedones, and cysts containing sebaceous matter and keratin. Systemic disease, including hepatitis, is a frequent complication.

Toxic hepatitis may also result from exposure to the fumes of hexachloronaphthalene, causing jaundice with nausea, abdominal discomfort, grayish or clay-colored stools, and dark urine. Deaths have occurred from long-term exposure.

Exposure–effect relationship

Repeated exposure to a mixture of penta- and hexachloronaphthalene at levels of $1.0\,mg/m^3$ may cause death due to severe liver injury.

Prognosis

Chloracne has been reported to persist for as long as 15 years after the complete cessation of exposure.

Differential diagnosis

Acute poisoning

Differential diagnosis of acute poisoning is not documented in the literature.

Chronic poisoning

Differentiate chloracne from acne vulgaris.

In cases of liver impairment, exclude other causes of liver parenchyma disorders, such as viral hepatitis and alcohol-related liver disease.

Susceptibility

Persons with liver disease and acne vulgaris are more sensitive to the effects of hexachloronaphthalene than others.

Health examinations

Preplacement examination

The preplacement health examination should include a medical history and a physical examination, with special attention to the skin and liver. Liver function tests should also be carried out.

Periodic examinations

In medical terms, the periodic examination is the same as the preplacement one. It is usually carried out once a year.

Case management

Remove the intoxicated individual from exposure, and, if necessary, immediately flush eyes and skin with water. Treat liver disease symptomatically. Chloracne should be treated appropriately.

Control measures

Technical control measures to reduce hexachloronaphthalene vapours in the workroom air should be applied. Skin contact should be avoided whenever possible. Protective clothing and good personal hygiene are essential preventive measures. Respirators are advisable when fumes are present. The exposure limit for hexachloronaphthalene has been set by various countries at $0.2\,mg/m^3$.

POLYCHLORINATED BIPHENYLS

Properties of the causal agents

Polychlorinated biphenyls (PCBs) are organochlorine compounds that have a molecular formula of $C_{12}H_{10-x}Cl_x$. Thus, 1–10 chlorine atoms may replace a corresponding number of hydrogen atoms. They range from clear, pale yellow liquids to viscous solids, their consistency increasing with their degree of chlorination. Their boiling points range from 325 °C to 366.11 °C.

Commercial polychlorinated biphenyl mixtures contain varying quantities of impurities, among which chlorinated dibenzofurans and chlorinated naphthalenes have been identified.

Production and uses

PCBs are produced by the chlorination of biphenyl with anhydrous chlorine in the presence of iron filings or a ferric chloride catalyst. PCBs are used in capacitors, transformers, synthetic rubber, plasticizers, flame retardants, and investment casting waxes.

Occupations involving exposure to PCBs

Electrical workers are usually at greatest risk.

Mechanism of action

Absorption

PCBs enter the body by inhalation in the form of vapours, and absorption takes place mainly through the lungs. Absorption through intact skin is also possible.

Biotransformation

Metabolites of PCBs include mono- and polyhydroxylated derivatives and dechlorinated derivatives. They are, to varying degrees, conjugated with glucuronic or sulfuric acids.

Excretion

Metabolites have been found in the faeces, urine, and milk of mammals. The less chlorinated biphenyl compounds are more readily metabolized than are the more highly chlorinated ones. As a consequence, some of the highly chlorinated compounds persist in the tissue, especially in fat, for many years.

Assessment of exposure

Environmental assessment

The method of choice is air sampling in the breathing zone (preferably by personal sampling) using cellulose membrane filters, followed by gas chromatographic analysis.

Biological assessment

The blood PCB concentration evaluated with reference to the duration of exposure may be used to compare different levels of occupational exposure. Several national surveys give PCB concentrations in blood of around 3.0 µg/litre and in adipose tissue of around 1 mg/kg of body weight or less. However, higher values have been reported from some countries.

Clinical effects

Acute poisoning

Systematic effects include anorexia, nausea, abdominal pain, and oedema of the face and hands.

Chronic poisoning

PCBs produce chloracne on the face, ears, neck, shoulders, arms, chest, and abdomen (especially around the umbilicus and on the scrotum). The skin becomes dry with intense pruritis, non-inflammatory comedones, and cysts containing sebaceous matter and keratin. Systemic disease, including hepatitis with hepatomegaly, digestive disturbances, haematuria, burning of the eyes, and impotence are frequent complications. These signs may be associated with an increase in serum concentrations of alanine aminotransferase, aspartate aminotransferase, gammaglutamyl transpeptidase, ornithine carbamoyl transferase, and triglycerides. Some of these changes have been attributed to the contaminants in PCBs.

Delayed effects

Animal feeding studies suggest that PCBs may cause liver cancer. However, mortality studies in man have shown no consistent pattern of cancer deaths related to PCB exposure, except for some evidence of a relationship between PCB exposure and malignant melanoma.

Exposure–effect relationship

Symptoms of PCB poisoning have been reported in workers after a minimum of 5 months and an average of 14 months of exposure to 0.1 mg of PCBs/m^3 of air.

Prognosis

If exposure is discontinued, the liver injury is usually reversible, but chloracne may persist for as long as 15 years.

Differential diagnosis

Exclude other causes of liver impairment such as infectious hepatitis and alcohol-related liver disease.

Susceptibility

Persons with pre-existing dermatitis or liver disease are more sensitive.

Health examinations

Preplacement examination

The preplacement examination should include a medical history and a physical examination, with special attention to the skin and liver. Liver function tests should also be carried out.

Periodic examination

In medical terms, the periodic examination is the same as the preplacement one. It is usually carried out once a year. Liver function tests and tests for plasma triglycerides should also be done.

Case management

Patients showing liver impairment and persistent chloracne should be removed from exposure and treated according to their symptoms.

Control measures

Technical control measures should be applied to reduce air pollution by PCBs. In order to prevent skin contact, workers should wear PCB-resistant clothing and equipment, including respirators. Exposure limits in different countries range from $0.5 \, mg/m^3$ to $1.0 \, mg/m^3$.

VINYL CHLORIDE

Properties of the causal agent

Vinyl chloride (C_2H_3Cl) is a colourless explosive, flammable gas.

Production and uses

Vinyl chloride may be produced either by hydrochlorination of acetylene or by halogenation of ethylene. It is mainly used as a chemical intermediate in the manufacture of polyvinyl chloride and other resins.

Occupations involving exposure to vinyl chloride

Polyvinyl resin makers, organic chemical synthesizers, and rubber makers are at greatest risk of exposure.

Mechanism of action

Absorption

Vinyl chloride is absorbed mainly through the lungs.

Biotransformation

A metabolite of vinyl chloride, rather than vinyl chloride itself, causes the toxic effects. Some of the absorbed vinyl chloride is excreted unchanged. A varying amount is metabolized by epoxidation, yielding chloroacetaldehyde. Further oxidation and conjugation are responsible for the metabolites in the urine.

Excretion

Some of the absorbed vinyl chloride is excreted through the lungs in exhaled air. The rest is excreted in the urine, partly unchanged and partly as metabolites.

Assessment of exposure

Environmental assessment

The following method is recommended for measuring the air concentration of vinyl chloride: Draw a known volume of air through two small tubes placed in series and containing activated carbon to adsorb the vinyl chloride. Extract vinyl chloride from the tubes with carbon disulfide and analyse the solution by gas chromatography and flame-ionization detector.

Biological assessment

There are no specific tests in common use.

Clinical effects

Acute poisoning

The primary effect of acute exposure is central nervous system depression.

Chronic poisoning

Chronic exposure in polyvinyl chloride reactor-vessel cleaners has caused acro-osteolysis (degeneration of the terminal phalanges). Raynaud's phenomenon was the first manifestation noted by the workers, suggesting that vascular changes precede those in bone. Radiographic findings include lytic lesions in the distal phalanges of the hands, in the styloid processes of the ulna and the radius, and in the sacroiliac joints. Other adverse effects of vinyl chloride include thrombocytopenia, splenomegaly, hepatomegaly, and fibrosis of the liver capsule.

Delayed effects

Angiosarcoma of the liver, a rare complication in vinyl chloride polymerization workers, appears to be related to some phase of vinyl chloride processing. Clinical features include weakness, pleuritic pain, abdominal pain, weight loss, gastrointestinal bleeding, hepatomegaly, and splenomegaly.

Exposure–effect relationship

Exposure to 52 mg of vinyl chloride per m³ of air for five minutes was seen to cause dizziness, light-headedness, nausea, and dulling of vision and auditory cues. Neither clinical changes nor abnormal neurological responses were found in 13 volunteers exposed for $7\frac{1}{2}$ hours to 1.3 g/m³, although exposure to a time-weighted-average concentration of 780 mg/m³ for a working lifetime caused abnormal liver function tests but no overt clinical disease.

Prognosis

Minor liver damage is probably reversible. The prognosis of acro-osteolysis is uncertain. Angiosarcoma is fatal.

Differential diagnosis

Acute poisoning

In cases of extreme exposure, exclude other causes of mental confusion.

Chronic poisoning

Exclude other causes of liver disease, particularly hepatitis and cirrhosis. Liver scanning may provide useful clues.

Susceptibility

Persons with pre-existing liver disease are more susceptible than others.

Health examinations

Preplacement examination

The preplacement examination should include a medical history and a physical examination, with special attention to the liver, spleen, kidneys, skin, connective tissues, and the pulmonary system. Liver function tests should also be carried out.

Periodic examination

In medical terms, the periodic examination is the same as the preplacement one. It should be carried out annually.

Case management

Remove the intoxicated individual from exposure. Treat liver disease and acro-osteolysis symptomatically.

Control measures

Whenever possible, reduce exposure by the use of enclosed systems. In areas where air concentrations of vinyl chloride are likely to be high, proper protective clothing should be worn in order to prevent skin contact with vinyl chloride or polyvinyl chloride residues. Since vinyl chloride may be carcinogenic, exposure levels should be kept as low as possible.

CHAPTER 18

Diseases caused by benzene and its toxic homologues

BENZENE

Properties of the causal agent

Benzene (C_6H_6) is a colourless, volatile liquid with a characteristic odour. It boils at 80.1 °C, and is highly flammable. Its vapours are explosive.

Production and uses

Benzene is produced by the distillation of coal or crude oil. It is used as a raw material in the production of many aromatic compounds, such as styrene, phenol, cyclohexane, and nitrobenzene, and certain drugs, pesticides, and detergents. Sometimes it is also used as an extraction solvent. It is present in solvents for waxes, resins, rubber, plastics, lacquers, paints, glues, etc. In recent years its use as a solvent has been limited or prohibited in many countries owing to its toxicity. Benzene may be present in gasoline (petrol), toluene, and xylene as an impurity.

Occupations involving exposure to benzene

The following workers are at greatest risk of exposure: petrochemical workers in benzene production; workers in the chemical industry and in laboratories using benzene; synthetic glue makers; users of synthetic glues in the manufacture of shoes, leather or rubber goods, and furniture; dye makers; printers (in rotogravure particularly); and paint sprayers.

Pathophysiology

Absorption

Benzene enters the body in the form of vapour by inhalation, and absorption takes place mainly through the lungs. About 40–60% of inhaled amount is retained. Limited absorption through intact skin is possible upon direct contact with the liquid.

Biotransformation

The main final metabolite is phenol, which is excreted in the urine conjugated with sulfuric or glucuronic acid. Minor amounts are metabolized to catechol, hydroquinone, carbon dioxide, and muconic acid. The first step in the oxidation of benzene is the formation of benzene epoxide by mixed-function oxidases in the liver.

Excretion

Part of the absorbed benzene is excreted unchanged—12–50% in the expired air and less than 1% in the urine. The average amount of eliminated phenol represents about 30% of the absorbed dose.

Assessment of exposure

Environmental assessment

In order to prevent acute exposure, detector tubes may be used to measure benzene concentrations before entering workrooms that may have high concentrations of benzene vapour in the air. For regular monitoring of exposure, the time-weighted average should be assessed either by area sampling in the breathing zone or, preferably, by personal sampling.

Biological assessment

Phenol in urine. Phenol is a normal component of urine, the average concentration being 9.5 ± 3.6 mg/litre standardized to a relative density of urine of 1.024. In occupationally unexposed persons, the concentration of phenol in urine depends mainly on its intake by food and, to a lesser extent, on individual variations in metabolism. In occupational exposure to benzene, the following exposure values have been suggested for individual phenol concentrations in urine determined immediately after the workshift:

—about 100 mg phenol/litre of urine indicates exposure of approximately 80 mg benzene/m^3 of air for 8 hours (concentration × time (CT) = 640);

—about 50 mg phenol/litre of urine indicates an exposure of approximately 32 mg benzene/m^3 of air for 8 hours (CT = 256);

—over 25 mg phenol/litre of urine indicates some exposure to benzene; and

—less than 10 mg phenol/litre of urine probably indicates an absence of significant exposure.[1]

Benzene in expired air. There is a direct relationship between the level of exposure (CT) and the concentration of benzene in expired air. By this method it is possible to detect exposure to concentrations of benzene in the air lower than those detectable by the phenol test. It should be pointed out, however, that the phenol test is more practicable.

Clinical effects

High concentrations of benzene vapour cause narcotic effects and slight irritation to the eyes and mucous membranes of the respiratory tract. Long-term exposure to lower concentrations may result in bone-marrow suppression and may also be associated with increased incidence of leukaemias. Liquid benzene has a defatting effect on the skin; hence, contact with it may cause dermatitis.

Acute poisoning

The main narcotic effects include: dizziness, headache, confusion, feeling of drunkeness, nausea, staggering gait, coma, and death due to respiratory arrest.

Chronic poisoning

The most significant toxic effect of benzene exposure is the insidious, and often irreversible, injury to bone marrow, which is probably due to its metabolite benzene epoxide. Individual suscept-ibility and haematological findings vary greatly. Classical changes are thrombocytopenia, leukopenia or anaemia, or a combination of these (pancytopenia). An irritative initial phase with increase in the number of blood elements may sometimes precede other symptoms. In continuing exposure, panmyelopathy or aplastic anaemia may develop. Other haematological changes are less consistent and need not be monitored routinely.

Workers exposed to benzene in concentrations sufficient to cause bone-marrow suppression may feel ill even if there are no haematolog-ical changes.

Delayed effects

Besides pancytopenia, leukaemias attributable to benzene exposure have been recognized. They are mostly non-lymphoid or myeloblastic

---

[1] International Workshop on Toxicology of Benzene, Paris: 9th–11th November 1976. *International archives of occupational and environmental health*, **41**: 65–76 (1978).

leukaemias; sometimes, however, aleukemic leukaemia and erythro-leukaemia may also be seen. There may be a latent period of several years between the cessation of exposure to benzene and the onset of leukaemia. Bone-marrow suppression may precede the development of leukaemia.

Exposure–effect relationship

Initial symptoms of acute poisoning have been observed after exposure to concentrations between $160 \, mg/m^3$ and $480 \, mg/m^3$ for 5 hours. A 30–60 min exposure to a concentration of $2.5 \, g/m^3$ may cause unconsciousness, and a 5–10 min exposure to $65 \, g/m^3$ may result in death.

A review of benzene toxicology suggests that there is a depressive action on bone marrow following long-term exposure to concentrations of benzene above about $70–100 \, mg/m^3$. Bone-marrow hypoplasia resulting from exposure to lower concentrations has not been proved with certainty, but systematic investigations of this exposure level are very few.

No similar exposure–effect relationship for leukaemia has been found. Leukaemia is more likely to occur if the exposure level is high enough to cause cytopenia. It has been reported that in workers exposed to concentrations of benzene of $450–2000 \, mg/m^3$, the incidence of leukaemias is at least twice that found in the general population.

Prognosis

The prognosis of pancytopenia is favourable in the majority of workers if they are removed early from benzene exposure, although some changes may last for several years.

Differential diagnosis

Acute poisoning

Exclude other causes of confused state or coma (mainly metabolic or central nervous system affections) and prove high-level benzene exposure (by measuring phenol in urine and benzene in breath).

Chronic poisoning

Exclude haematological diseases known to have no relation to benzene toxicity and secondary cytopenias of known origin. Specialized haematological examinations and tests are usually necessary. Idiopathic cytopenias and leukaemias are clinically indistinguishable from those caused by exposure to benzene. A documented history of exposure is essential for assessing the probability of occupational origin, which increases when: (*a*) the exposure level is high enough to cause cytopenia; (*b*) leukaemia is preceded by myelopathy; and (*c*) abnormal cellular clones are present.

Susceptibility

Pregnant women (risk of abortion supposed) and those suffering from haematological diseases and chronic diseases that impair hepatic or renal functions related to benzene metabolism are more susceptible than others.

Health examinations

The main purpose of the health examination is to detect signs of bone marrow suppression while it is still at an early reversible stage and to uncover general contraindications to working with benzene.

Preplacement examination

The preplacement examination should include a medical history, a physical examination, and a blood count, including determination of blood platelets and a differential leukocyte count.

Periodic examinations

In medical terms, the periodic examination is the same as the preplacement one. Since little is known about the relationship between the level of exposure and the average time at which first haematological signs appear, an interval of one year between medical examinations is recommended, provided the hygienic conditions at the workplace are satisfactory (i.e. the exposure limit is not exceeded).

Screening test

If high exposure levels are detected at a workplace, the blood count determinations should be repeated at intervals of 3–6 months.

Case management

Patients suffering from chronic benzene poisoning must be removed from further exposure to benzene. There is no specific treatment, but therapies for other blood diseases of similar type, may be used.

Control measures

ILO Convention No. 136 (1971) and Recommendation No. 144 (1971) apply to all industrial activities entailing exposure to benzene and products, the benzene content of which exceeds 1% by volume. Less harmful substitutes should be used instead of benzene. Exposure should be limited by: (a) enclosing hazardous systems so far as practicable; (b) providing exhaust ventilation to remove benzene vapour to the extent necessary; and (c) using personal protection devices against respiratory or skin absorption.

Exposure limits for benzene in different countries range from $5 \, mg/m^3$ to $80 \, mg/m^3$. Since benzene is a carcinogen, exposure to it should be kept as low as possible.

TOLUENE

Properties of the causal agent

Toluene ($C_6H_5CH_3$) is a volatile, colourless liquid with a characteristic odour. It boils at 110.6 °C, is flammable, and its vapours are explosive.

Production and uses

Toluene is produced mainly from crude oil. It is used as a raw material for the synthesis of compounds such as saccharin, chloramine-T, trinitrotoluene (TNT), toluene diisocyanate, and many dyestuffs. It is also used as a solvent for rubber, tar, asphalt, and cellulose paints and varnishes.

Occupations involving exposure to toluene

Petrochemical workers in toluene production, workers in the chemical industry or laboratories using toluene as a raw material or solvent, dye makers and paint workers are at greatest risk.

Pathophysiology

Absorption

Toluene is absorbed mainly through the inhalation of its vapour. Limited skin absorption is possible through direct contact with the liquid. About 40–60% of the inhaled amount is retained in the body.

Biotransformation

About 60–80% is metabolized into benzoic acid, which then conjugates with glycine to form hippuric acid.

Excretion

About 20% of the absorbed toluene is exhaled. Hippuric acid is rapidly eliminated in urine (almost entirely in 24 hours).

Assessment of exposure

Environmental assessment

In order to prevent acute exposure, detector tubes may be used to measure toluene concentrations before entering workrooms that may have high concentrations of toluene vapour in the air. For regular monitoring of exposure, the time weighted average should be assessed, either by area sampling in the breathing zone or, preferably, by personal sampling.

Biological assessment

The measurement of hippuric acid in urine is the most important method. In subjects not exposed to toluene, the concentration of hippuric acid, originating mainly from food containing benzoic acid or benzoates, rarely exceeds 0.947 mol per mol of creatinine (1.5 g/g). An average of about 1.58 mol of hippuric acid per mol creatinine (2.5 g/g) in urine collected from groups of workers at the end of the workshift corresponds to an exposure level of 375 mg of toluene/m^3 of air for 8 hours; 0.947 mol of hippuric acid per mol of creatinine (1.5 g/g) corresponds to about 200 mg of toluene/m^3 of air.

Clinical effects

The narcotic and neurotoxic properties of toluene represent the main health hazards. There is no convincing evidence of damage to other organs. Toluene is not haematotoxic.

Acute poisoning

The signs of acute poisoning include dizziness, drowsiness, and unconsciousness. Death due to respiratory arrest is possible.

Chronic poisoning

The chief complaints relate to its narcotic action. They include: headache, lassitude, general weakness, impairment of coordination and memory, nausea, anorexia. Objective signs of lesions of the central, peripheral, and autonomic nervous systems are found far less often. Menstrual dysfunction in women following toluene exposure has been reported.

Exposure–effect relationship

The initial symptoms of acute poisoning have been observed in experimental exposures of volunteers at levels of about $750\,mg/m^3$ for 8 hours or $1125\,mg/m^3$ for 20 min. Chronic poisoning has been reported to occur at about 200–$400\,mg/m^3$ (time-weighted average).

Prognosis

The prognosis of toluene poisoning is favourable.

Differential diagnosis

Acute poisoning

Exclude other causes of confused state or coma (mainly metabolic or central nervous system affections), and confirm high-level exposure to toluene by measuring hippuric acid in urine, toluene in breath, and toluene vapour concentration in the workroom air.

Chronic poisoning

Exclude neurological and psychiatric diseases. Evidence of high-level exposure (environmental and biological assessment) must be present. Specialized neurological, psychiatric, and psychological examinations may be necessary.

Susceptibility

Chronic diseases of the central nervous system and hepatic or renal function impairments increase susceptibility.

Health examinations

Preplacement examination

The preplacement examination should include a medical history and a physical examination.

Periodic examination

In medical terms, the periodic examination is the same as the preplacement one. It should be carried out every 2–3 years depending on the level of exposure.

Case management

The patient should be kept away from exposure until he recovers. There is no specific treatment.

Control measures

Exposure should be controlled by enclosing processes generating toluene vapours. Personal protective devices against respiratory or skin absorption should be used whenever necessary.

Exposure limits in different countries range from $50 \, mg/m^3$ to $375 \, mg/m^3$. According to a WHO Study Group,[1] the health-based exposure limit for toluene may be in the range of 200–375 mg/m³.

XYLENE

Properties of the causal agent

Xylene $(C_6H_4(CH_3)_2)$ is a colourless volatile liquid with a typical aromatic odour. It boils at 140°C and is flammable. The commercial product is a mixture of three isomers ortho-, meta- and para-, with *m*-xylene predominating (usually 60–70%).

Production and uses

Xylene is produced mainly from crude oil. It is widely used as a substrate for organic synthesis and thinner for paints and lacquers. It is a constituent of aviation fuel.

Occupations involving exposure to xylene

Petrochemical workers in xylene production, workers in the chemical industry or laboratories using xylene as a raw material or solvent, and paint and printing (rotogravure) workers are at greatest risk of exposure.

---

[1] WHO Technical Report Series, No. 664, 1981.

Mechanism of action

Absorption

Xylene is absorbed mainly through the inhalation of its vapour. Skin absorption is possible through direct contact with the liquid. About 40–60% of the total inhaled amount is retained in the body.

Biotransformation

About 95% of the absorbed xylene is metabolized almost entirely to methylbenzoic acid, which then conjugates with glycine to form methylhippuric acid.

Excretion

The elimination of the unchanged xylene in exhaled air and of its metabolites (methylhippuric acids) in urine is rapid and reaches completion within 18 hours after the termination of exposure.

Assessment of exposure

Environmental assessment

In order to prevent acute exposure, detector tubes may be used to measure xylene concentrations before entering workrooms that may have high concentrations of xylene vapour in the air. For regular monitoring of exposure, the time-weighted average should be assessed either by area sampling in the breathing zone or, preferably, by personal sampling.

Biological assessment

Measurement of methylhippuric acid in urine is the most important method. It has been estimated that an 8-hour exposure to 200 mg of xylene/m^3 of air corresponds to a methylhippuric acid concentration in the urine of about 0.00725 mol/litre (1.4 g/litre) on the basis of samples collected from groups of workers at the end of a workshift, corrected to a relative density of urine of 1.024.

Clinical effects

The narcotic properties of xylene represent the main health hazard. There is no convincing evidence of damage to other organs.

Acute poisoning

The signs of acute poisoning include dizziness, drowsiness, and unconsciousness. Death due to respiratory arrest is possible.

Chronic poisoning

Complaints of headache, irritability, fatigue, lassitude, dyspeptic disorders, sleepiness during the day and sleep disorders at night have been reported. Objective signs of impairment of the nervous system are found far less often.

Exposure–effect relationship

Impairment of reaction time was observed in volunteers exposed to 870 mg/m^3 for 3 hours. There are no sufficient data on long-term exposure.

Prognosis

The prognosis of xylene poisoning is favourable.

Differential diagnosis

Acute poisoning

Exclude other causes of confused state or coma (mainly metabolic and central nervous system affections) and confirm high-level exposure to xylene by measuring methylhippuric acid in urine, xylene in breath, and xylene vapour concentrations in the workroom air.

Chronic poisoning

Exclude neurological and psychiatric diseases. Evidence of high-level exposure (environmental and biological assessment) must be present. Specialized neurological, psychiatric, and psychological examinations may be necessary.

Susceptibility

Pregnant women (teratogenic effects observed in animals), and those suffering from chronic diseases of the central nervous system or diseases impairing hepatic or renal functions are more susceptible than others.

Health examinations

Preplacement examination

The preplacement examination should include a medical history and a physical examination.

Periodic examination

In medical terms, the periodic examination is the same as the preplacement one. It should be carried out every 2–3 years.

Case management

The patient should be kept away from exposure until he recovers. There is no specific treatment.

Control measures

Exposure should be controlled by using enclosed systems. Exposure limits should be respected. Personal protective devices against respiratory or skin absorption should be used whenever necessary.

Exposure limits in different countries range from $50 \, mg/m^3$ to $435 \, mg/m^3$.

CHAPTER 19

Diseases caused by toxic nitro and amino derivatives of benzene and its homologues

The toxic nitro and amino derivatives of benzene and its homologues constitute a large and varied group of compounds of great commercial importance that have similar toxicological characteristics. The simplest of these derivatives are aniline and nitrobenzene, both of which are discussed below as examples. These derivatives of benzene and its homologues and analogues differ toxicologically from their parent compounds, such as benzene, toluene, xylene, and naphthalene.

ANILINE

Properties of the causal agent

Aniline ($C_6H_5NH_2$) is a colourless to pale yellow oily liquid with an aromatic amine-like odour.

Production and uses

The most common method of production is the catalytic hydrogenation of nitrobenzene at a temperature of 250–300 °C under a pressure slightly above atmospheric. Aniline is used in the manufacture of dyes, rubber accelerators and antioxidants, pharmaceuticals, resins, varnishes, perfumes, and shoe polish. It is also used as a solvent and as a vulcanizing agent in rubber manufacture.

Occupations involving exposure to aniline

Chemical and rubber workers, dye makers, and vulcanizers are at greatest risk.

Mechanism of action

Absorption

Aniline vapour is absorbed mainly through the lungs. Slow absorption of vapour through the skin is also possible. Liquid aniline is readily absorbed through intact skin, often from contaminated clothes, gloves, and shoes.

Biotransformation

About 15–60 % of the absorbed aniline is oxidized to p-aminophenol, which is excreted in the urine as glucuronide and sulfate conjugates. The intermediate metabolite, phenyl hydroxylamine, is apparently responsible for certain toxic effects of aniline (methaemoglobinaemia).

Excretion

Aniline is not found in the expired air. Less than 1 % of the absorbed dose is excreted unchanged in the urine. In exposed workers, the urinary p-aminophenol concentration appears to be directly related to the blood methaemoglobin concentration.

Assessment of exposure

Environmental assessment

The measurement of aniline vapour concentrations in workrooms, preferably by personal sampling and gas chromatographic analysis, is the method of choice.

Biological assessment

The method of choice is the measurement of p-aminophenol in urine. The following relationships between aniline exposure and p-aminophenol in urine have been observed:

- an 8-hour exposure to 5 mg of aniline/m^3 of air results in 35 mg of p-aminophenol being excreted in the urine within the first 24 hours following exposure;
- an 8-hour exposure to 19 mg of aniline/m^3 of air results in 150 mg of p-aminophenol in urine in 24 hours;
- at the above two exposure levels, the rates of p-aminophenol excretion in urine during the fourth and sixth hour of exposure are 1.5 mg/hour and 13 mg/hour, respectively.

Note that this test is nonspecific for aniline because certain other aromatic compounds are also metabolized to the same end-product (i.e., *p*-aminophenol). The use of the analgesic phenacetin also leads to *p*-aminophenol in urine.

Another indicator of over-exposure to aniline is elevated methaemoglobin concentration in blood, the normal level of which does not exceed 1.5 g per 100 g haemoglobin.

Clinical effects

Aniline absorption causes anoxia owing to the formation of methaemoglobin.

Acute poisoning

The development of methaemoglobinaemia is often insidious. Following skin absorption, the onset of symptoms may be delayed for up to 4 hours. Headache is commonly the first symptom and may become quite intense as the severity of methaemoglobinaemia progresses. Cyanosis occurs when the blood level of methaemoglobin exceeds 15 g per 100 g haemoglobin. Blueness develops first in the lips, then in the nose and the earlobes. The individual usually feels well, has no complaints, and insists that nothing is wrong until the methaemoglobin level approaches approximately 40 g per 100 g haemoglobin. Above this level, there is usually weakness and dizziness; at up to 70 g per 100 g haemoglobin there may be ataxia, dyspnoea on mild exertion, and tachycardia. Coma may ensue above 70 g/100 g and the lethal level is estimated at 85–90 g/100 g haemoglobin. Erythrocytic inclusions (Heinz bodies) develop in serious poisonings, but haemolysis is rare.

Liquid aniline is mildly irritating to the eyes.

Chronic poisoning

Although liver damage and cerebral effects from repeated exposure to aniline have been alleged, the general view is that there are no chronic effects.

Exposure–effect relationship

Exposure lasting several hours to aniline vapour at about 25–200 mg/m³ causes mild symptoms. Exposure to concentrations in excess of about 400–600 mg/m³ for one hour causes serious methaemoglobinaemia. Skin absorption of the liquid, and possibly of the vapour, should not be overlooked.

Prognosis

Occasional deaths in severe acute poisoning have been reported, but effects are generally regarded as reversible and without residual damage.

Differential diagnosis

Acute poisoning

Exclude other causes of cyanosis such as hypoxia due to cardiopulmonary disease. In judging the significance of *p*-aminophenol concentration in urine, ascertain that it is not due to overdoses of nitrites, acetanilide, phenacetin, sulfonamides and other similar drugs. Exclude any hereditary haemoglobinopathies.

Chronic poisoning

The differential diagnosis of chronic poisoning is not documented in the literature. However, there may be haematological effects in susceptible individuals (see also Chapter 32).

Susceptibility

Individuals with hereditary haemoglobinopathy and any congenital heart disease causing hypoxia, are more susceptible than others.

Health examinations

Preplacement examination

The preplacement examination should include a medical history and a physical examination, with special attention to the cardiovascular system, lungs, and blood. Special attention should be paid to the possibility of hypersusceptibility to methaemoglobinaemia.

Periodic examinations

In medical terms, the periodic examination is the same as the preplacement one. It is usually carried out once a year.

Case management

All aniline on the body must be removed. Immediately remove and discard all clothing, gloves, and footwear. Wash the whole body (from head to toe) with soap and water. Pay special attention to hair and scalp, finger and toenails, nostrils, and ear canals. Administer oxygen to alleviate the headache and general sense of weakness and confine the patient to bed. Determine the methaemoglobin concentration in the blood every 3–6 hours for 18–24 hours. Repeat skin cleansing if the methaemoglobin concentration appears to rise after 3–4 hours. Ascorbic acid (administered intravenously) and methylene blue have been used for reducing methaemoglobinaemia; methylene blue should be used with caution and in severe cases only. In the case of eye irritation, flush the eyes with water.

Control measures

Skin contact must be avoided by the use of protective clothing, including impervious boots and gloves. All workers should know how to recognize the early signs of cyanosis (blueness of the nose, lips, earlobes) in fellow workers. Appropriate ventilation should be provided for the control of aniline vapour, and where aniline is handled at elevated temperatures, either enclosed processes should be used or very effective ventilation should be provided.

Exposure limits for aniline in different countries range from 0.1 mg/m^3 to 19 mg/m^3.

NITROBENZENE

Properties of the causal agent

Nitrobenzene ($C_6H_5NO_2$) is a colourless oily liquid that turns yellow on exposure to air. It has an odour of bitter almonds.

Uses

Nitrobenzene is used in the manufacture of dyes and explosives and as a chemical intermediate and solvent.

Occupations involving exposure to nitrobenzene

Chemical workers and dye makers are at greatest risk of exposure.

Mechanism of action

Absorption

Nitrobenzene vapour is absorbed with 80% efficiency through the lungs. Slow absorption of the vapour through the skin is also possible. Liquid nitrobenzene is readily absorbed through intact skin.

Biotransformation

Nitrobenzene is metabolized by both oxidation and reduction; the former leads to the formation of *p*-nitrophenol and the latter gives rise to aniline, which is further oxidized to *p*-aminophenol.

Excretion

About 13–16% of the absorbed dose is excreted in the urine as *p*-nitrophenol and probably less than 10% as *p*-aminophenol. Both are eliminated as sulfate or glucuronide conjugates.

Assessment of exposure

Environmental assessment

The measurement of nitrobenzene vapour concentrations in workrooms, preferably by personal sampling and gas chromatographic analysis is the method of choice.

Biological assessment

The measurement of *p*-nitrophenol in urine at the end of the workshift is the method of choice. It has been estimated that 5 mg of nitrobenzene/m^3 of air may result in about 1.5–5.5 mg *p*-nitrophenol per litre of urine. The measurement of methaemoglobin in blood (normal level up to 1.5 g per 100 g haemoglobin) may also prove to be a useful method of assessing exposure.

Clinical effects

Nitrobenzene causes anoxia owing to the formation of methaemoglobin in the blood.

Acute poisoning

Signs and symptoms of overexposure result from the loss of oxygen-carrying capacity of the blood. The onset of the symptoms of methaemoglobinaemia is often insidious and may be delayed by up to four hours. Headache is commonly the first symptom and may become quite intense as the severity of methaemoglobinaemia progresses. Cyanosis develops early in the course of intoxication and is characterized by blueness of the lips, nose, and earlobes; it is usually recognized first by fellow workers and occurs when the methaemoglobin level is 15 g/100 g haemoglobin or more. The individual usually feels well, has no complaints, and insists that nothing is wrong with him until the methaemoglobin level approaches 40 g/100 g. At methaemoglobin levels ranging from 40 g to 70 g per 100 g haemo-globin there is headache, weakness, dizziness, ataxia, dyspnoea on mild exertion, tachycardia, nausea, vomiting, and drowsiness. Coma may ensue when the methaemoglobin level rises above 70 g/100 g. The lethal level of methaemoglobin is estimated at 85–90 g/100 g haemog-lobin. Erythrocytic inclusion (Heinz bodies) may develop in severe poisoning, but haemolysis is rare. Nitrobenzene is mildly irritating to the eyes. It may produce dermatitis due to primary irritation or sensitization.

Chronic poisoning

Reversible anaemia, liver damage, and peripheral neuropathy have been reported to result from long-term exposure.

Exposure–effects relationship

Exposure of workers to 200 mg of nitrobenzene per m³ of air for 6 months resulted in some cases of intoxication and anaemia. Concentrations ranging between 15 mg/m³ and 30 mg/m³ caused headache and vertigo. Increased methaemoglobin and sulfhaemoglobin levels and Heinz bodies were observed in the blood in both cases.

Prognosis

The effects of methaemoglobinaemia are generally regarded as acute and promptly reversible. Severe exposures may produce more lasting effects on the blood, liver, and the nervous system.

Differential diagnosis

Acute poisoning

Exclude other causes of cyanosis including that from drugs, cardiopulmonary disease, and haemoglobinopathies.

Chronic poisoning

Exclude other causes of anaemia, liver damage, neuropathies, and sensitization dermatitis.

Susceptibility

Hereditary haemoglobinopathies, congenital heart disease causing cyanosis, chronic alcoholism, and higher ambient temperatures are said to increase susceptibility.

Health examinations

Preplacement examination

The preplacement examination should include a medical history and a physical examination, with special attention to the cardiovascular system, lungs, and blood. Hereditary haemoglobinopathy should be identified.

Periodic examination

In medical terms, the periodic examination is the same as the preplacement one. In addition, determinations of haemoglobin and haematocrit and liver function tests should be carried out, usually once a year.

Case management

All nitrobenzene on the body must be removed. Immediately remove and discard all clothing, gloves, and footwear. Wash the whole body (from head to toe) with soap and water. Pay special attention to the hair and scalp, the finger and toenails, nostrils, and ear canals. Give oxygen to alleviate the headache and general sense of weakness and confine the patient to bed. Determine the methaemoglobin level in the blood every 3–6 hours for 18–24 hours. Repeat skin cleansing if the methaemoglobin level appears to rise after 3–4 hours. In general, patients will return to normal within 24 hours, provided all sources of further absorption are completely eliminated. Ascorbic acid (administered intravenously) and methylene blue have been used for reducing methaemoglobinaemia; methylene blue should be used with caution and in severe cases only. In the case of eye irritation, flush the eyes with water.

Control measures

Adequate ventilation of workrooms is essential if the processes are not fully enclosed. Personal protective devices including respiratory masks, eyewear, protective clothing, and impervious gloves and shoes should be used whenever necessary.

The exposure time of each worker may be limited by job rotation. In order to avoid skin absorption, a high standard of personal hygiene should be enforced, with emphasis on hot showers (using soap) and daily change of work clothes.

Exposure limits for nitrobenzene in different countries range from 3 mg/m^3 to 10 mg/m^3.

CHAPTER 20

Diseases caused by nitroglycerin and other nitric acid esters

Properties of the causal agents

The most important representatives of this group are nitroglycerin and ethylene glycol dinitrate. Nitroglycerin (glyceryl trinitrate: $C_3H_5(ONO_2)_3$) is a pale yellow, explosive, oily liquid with a sweetish odour. Ethylene glycol dinitrate ($C_2H_4O_2(NO_2)_2$) is a yellowish odourless liquid.

Production and uses

Nitroglycerin and ethylene glycol dinitrate are produced by the nitration of glycerol and glycol, respectively. Both are used in the manufacture of explosives and rocket propellants; nitroglycerin is also used in medicine as a vasodilator.

Occupations involving exposure to nitroglycerin and ethylene glycol dinitrate

Workers engaged in the production of these substances and in the manufacture and use of explosives (e.g., in mines) are at greatest risk of exposure. Workers handling these substances in the pharmaceutical industry may also be at risk.

Mechanism of action

Absorption

Both compounds are rapidly absorbed through the lungs, skin, and the digestive tract.

Biotransformation

Nitroglycerin and ethyl glycol dinitrate are metabolized mainly in the liver. First, they react with reduced glutathion in the presence of certain enzymes that act as catalysts. This reaction yields inorganic

142

nitrites. In a further reaction the inorganic nitrites are oxidized to nitrates and these compounds are excreted in the urine. Metabolism by direct hydrolysis is also possible.

Excretion

All absorbed nitroglycerin is eliminated in the form of metabolites: carbon dioxide, dinitro- and mononitroglycerin, glycerol, etc. About 60 % of ethylene glycol dinitrate is excreted in the urine in the form of inorganic nitrates; about 0.5 % is excreted as mononitroglycol. Partly denitrated metabolites may be conjugated with glucuronic acid and excreted in the urine as glucuronides.

Assessment of exposure

Environmental assessment

The concentrations of nitroesters in the air of workplaces may not reflect the actual level of occupational exposure since higher absorption may result from percutaneous exposure than from inhalation.

Biological assessment

Although the determination of nitroesters in blood and of inorganic nitrates in urine is possible, the levels are not reliable reflections of exposure.

Clinical effects

Nitroesters and the intermediates of ethylene glycol dinitrate metabolism (mononitroglycol and nitrites) cause vasodilatation with a subsequent fall in blood pressure, heart rate acceleration, and pulse pressure reduction. After the first contact with nitroesters, or on resuming work after a long period of rest, the worker may develop headache, nausea, weakness, and palpitations and may even collapse. Physical examinations of such patients reveal a weak accelerated pulse and decreased blood pressure. After daily repeated exposures most workers acquire a tolerance, and the fall in blood pressure is less. This is not due to changes in metabolism but to the physiological regulatory mechanisms. However, there may be a decreased tolerance to alcohol, digestive troubles, sleep disturbances, paresthesias, tremor, and mental inhibition.

After prolonged exposure, anginal precordial pain may appear at the end of the weekend or vacations. This pain is often referred to as "Monday morning angina". It is not provoked by exertion, which is the case with angina in ischaemic heart disease, but comes on at rest. Not all patients are relieved by the administration of nitroglycerin.

The electrocardiogram may exceptionally show some transitory changes. There is still no explanation for the cases of sudden death occurring after the discontinuation (e.g., on holidays) of exposure to a mixture of nitroesters. This dramatic termination of prolonged exposure is primarily attributed to the action of ethylene glycol dinitrate. However, cases of sudden death have also been reported after exposure to nitroglycerin. It is assumed that death is caused by ventricular fibrillation in association with an increase in the activity of the sympathetic nervous system. Autopsy seldom reveals athero-sclerotic or thrombotic occlusion of coronary arteries.

After a job transfer, attacks of angina-like pain usually diminish or disappear completely. Carcinogenic or teratogenic effects of nitroesters have not been demonstrated.

Differential diagnosis

Headache, nausea, weakness, or collapse may be the first nonspecific symptoms of many diseases. Chest pain may be a symptom of coronary heart disease or of disease of the vertebral column, and digestive, neurological and psychiatric disorders may also result from nontoxic causes.

Susceptibility

Cardiovascular diseases and disorders of the central and autonomic nervous systems (particularly vasomotor regulation) and of the digestive tract and liver increase susceptibility.

Health examinations

Preplacement examination

The preplacement examination should include a medical history and a physical examination, with special attention to the cardiovascular and nervous systems and liver and psychiatric disorders. In addition, an electrocardiogram at rest and after exertion should be taken.

Periodic examination

In medical terms, the periodic examination is the same as the preplacement one and it is usually carried out once a year. In addition, an electrocardiogram should be taken at the time when precordial pain occurs.

Case management

Workers with repeated episodes of unconsciousness, collapse, or precordial pain should be removed from exposure.

Control measures

The exposure limits established in some countries range between 0.2 mg/m³ and 5.0 mg/m³ for nitroglycerin, and between 0.2 mg/m³ and 1.2 mg/m³ for ethylene glycol dinitrate. Safety measures include the provision of protective clothing to all workers, in order to prevent absorption through the skin, and the installation of appropriate ventilation. The National Institute of Occupational Health and Safety in the United States of America has recommended that the concentrations of nitroglycerin and ethylene glycol dinitrate in air should be kept lower than the level at which they cause vasodilatation (0.1 mg/m³). It is expected that this will reduce the risk of cardiac complications. [1]

---

[1] NATIONAL INSTITUTE OF OCCUPATIONAL HEALTH. *Occupational exposure to nitroglycerine and ethylene glycol dinitrate.* Washington, DC, Department of Health, Education, and Welfare, 1978.

CHAPTER 21

Diseases caused by alcohols, glycols, and ketones

ALCOHOLS AND GLYCOLS

Properties of the causal agents

Alcohols are hydrocarbons with a hydrogen atom replaced by one hydroxyl (OH) group and glycols are hydrocarbons with two hydroxyl groups. Short- and medium-chain alcohols are liquids, and some of them (methyl alcohol and ethyl alcohol) are highly volatile. Glycols are viscous liquids with low volatility and a sweetish odour.

Uses

Alcohols and glycols are used in various industrial processes including: (a) the syntheses of other organic compounds; (b) as solvents for pigments, resins, paints, inks and plastics; (c) in cutting oils; (d) as antifreeze fluids; (e) in the production of certain foods, drugs, and cosmetics; and (f) in the textile, rubber, and plastics industries. The most commonly used alcohols are methyl, ethyl, propyl, n-butyl and amyl alcohol. Ethylene and propylene glycol derivatives of industrial importance include ethers (ethylene glycol monomethyl ether and ethylene glycol monoethyl ether), esters (ethylene glycol acetate), ether–esters (ethylene glycol monomethyl ether acetate) and polyglycols. These compounds are extensively used as hydraulic fluids and as solvents for a variety of materials.

Occupations involving exposure to alcohols and glycols

Workers in the production or use of these substances, dye makers, dyers, printers, etc. are at greatest risk of exposure.

Mechanism of action

Absorption

In occupational exposure, alcohols, glycols, and their derivatives enter the body by either inhalation or transcutaneous absorption.

146

While highly volatile alcohols such as methyl and ethyl alcohols are mainly absorbed through the lungs, glycols are absorbed mostly through the skin. Accidental poisoning may result from ingestion of these compounds.

The distribution of these compounds in the body is related to the water content of the tissues; methyl alcohol and its metabolites accumulate selectively in the cerebrospinal and ocular fluids, causing pronounced local effects.

Biotransformation

The metabolic transformation of alcohols and glycols involves progressive oxidation of the hydroxyl group(s) to the corresponding aldehydes and carboxylic acids. Methyl alcohol is metabolized into formic acid, ethyl alcohol into acetaldehyde and acetic acid, and ethylene glycol into glycolic, glyoxylic, and oxalic acids.

Excretion

The metabolites, whether free or conjugated, are excreted in the urine. Volatile compounds are partly eliminated in exhaled air.

Assessment of exposure

Environmental assessment

High airborne concentrations can be easily detected by smell, but sensitivity is lost with continued exposure. Assessment of exposure may be performed by air sampling and analysis in the breathing zone or by personal sampling. However, it should be pointed out that with this procedure one cannot assess the risk of skin absorption.

Biological assessment

There are no reliable routine methods for biological monitoring. The final metabolites in urine or volatile alcohols in expired air could be measured, but the exact relationship between exposure level and amounts excreted is unknown.

Clinical effects

Under normal occupational exposure conditions, alcohols and glycols do not pose any major health hazards. They cause irritation of the skin and mucous membranes and have narcotic effects on the central nervous system. Because of its slow elimination, prolonged high-level exposure to methyl alcohol may cause optic nerve damage.

Acute poisoning

Acute poisoning from alcohols and glycols in industry is rare and occurs mainly as a result of accidental ingestion. Acutely intoxicated patients complain of headache, vertigo, confusion, feeling of drunkenness, nausea, vomiting, epigastric pain, and sensory function impairment. Methyl alcohol poisoning also produces visual disturbances due to optic retrobulbar neuritis, which may progress to optic atrophy. Metabolic acidosis due to the formation of formic acid is the typical biochemical feature of acute methyl alcohol poisoning.

Central nervous system depression, nausea, vomiting, and abdominal pain are the early manifestations of acute ethylene glycol poisoning. However, respiratory and cardiac failure may occur within a short time and the last stage of intoxication is dominated by renal failure with oliguria, proteinuria, and large amounts of oxalate crystals in the urinary sediment.

Acute exposure to glycol ethers and esters may result in marked narcotic effects and encephalopathy; pulmonary oedema and toxic effects on the kidney and liver are also possible.

Chronic poisoning

Except for occasional headache and upper respiratory tract irritation, no typical syndromes are usually associated with chronic exposure. Eye and upper respiratory tract irritation, optic neuritis with photophobia and disturbed vision, and central nervous system disorders are the manifestations of chronic methyl alcohol intoxication.

Ethyl alcohol intake may lead to the induction of hepatic microsomal enzymes and may alter the biotransformation rate of drugs and other exogenous substances.

Delayed effects

Workers employed in the production of isopropyl alcohol by the strong acid process exhibit an increased incidence of paranasal sinus neoplasms caused by the active intermediates and/or by-products associated with this type of synthesizing process. No such risk occurs with the manufacture of isopropyl alcohol by other processes or with its use.

Exposure–effect relationship

In general, concentrations in the range of some hundreds of mg/m³ of air may induce irritation of eyes or mucosae or narcotic effects.

Prognosis

If properly treated, the prognosis of acute poisoning is favourable. Optic neuritis from methyl alcohol may result in permanent vision impairment or blindness.

Differential diagnosis

Acute poisoning must be distinguished from other causes of states of confusion or coma, particularly those of metabolic origin or affections of the cardiovascular or central nervous system. Acidosis and optic neuritis are characteristic of methyl alcohol poisoning as are renal failure and oxalate crystal elimination of ethylene glycol poisoning. It is essential to obtain evidence of a high level of exposure at the workplace.

Susceptibility

Individuals with pre-existing impairment of the nervous system, alcoholics, those suffering from chronic liver and kidney diseases and those undergoing drug treatment for chronic illnesses are more susceptible than others.

Health examinations

Preplacement examination

The preplacement examination should include a medical history and a physical examination, with special attention to the nervous system.

Periodic examination

In medical terms the periodic examination is the same as the pre-placement one. The examinations should be annual if the hygienic conditions at the workplace are satisfactory. At higher levels of exposure or when acute or subacute poisoning is possible, medical examinations should be more frequent. Besides a general medical evaluation, an examination of the central nervous system and liver and kidney tests may also be required. In the case of methyl alcohol exposure, visual performance should be regularly tested.

Case management

There is no specific treatment for exposure to alcohols and glycols. Intensive care, correction of acidosis and general supportive measures are recommended for treating acute intoxications.

Control measures

Industrial exposure to alcohols and glycols and their derivatives can be controlled without difficulty by observing good general hygiene in the workplace. When highly volatile compounds are used adequate ventilation is essential. Absorption through the skin can be prevented by the wearing of gloves and appropriate protective clothing. When concentrations are expected to rise (e.g., in heating or spraying operations), personal protective equipment to prevent eye and skin contact and efficient respiratory protection are strongly recommended.

Different countries have the following exposure limits for alcohols and glycols:

Alcohols. Methyl alcohol 50–260 mg/m³, ethyl alcohol 200–2000 mg/m³, *n*-propyl alcohol 200–500 mg/m³, butyl alcohol 10–200 mg/m³, amyl alcohol 10–300 mg/m³.

Glycols. Ethylene glycol 100–260 mg/m³, ethylene glycol monoethyl ether 40–80 mg/m³.

KETONES

Properties of the causal agents

Ketones are aliphatic or aromatic compounds characterized by the presence of the carbonyl (C = O) group. They are colourless liquids, moderately to highly volatile, and have a typical aromatic odour. The best known ketone is acetone (dimethylketone), followed by butanone (methyl ethyl ketone).

Production and uses

Ketones are commercially produced by catalytic dehydrogenation or oxidation of secondary alcohols, which are usually derived from hydration of olefins in the petrochemical industry.

Ketones have numerous industrial applications. They are used as solvents for oils, cellulose esters, resins, pigments, dyes, inks, adhesives, paints, and lacquers. They are important chemical agents in the manufacture of synthetic rubber, lubricating oils, artificial leather, paints, varnishes, perfumes, and cosmetics. They are also used as cleaning agents.

Occupations involving exposure to ketones

Workers in the production of ketones and those in the above-mentioned industries are at greatest risk.

Mechanism of action

Absorption

In industrial exposure, the major route of absorption is by the inhalation of vapour. Absorption through intact skin may also become significant after extensive contact with liquid ketones.

Biotransformation

Ketones are metabolized in the body by the mixed-function oxidase system, producing oxidized derivatives. The metabolic pathways of methyl n-butyl ketone (2-hexanone) and n-hexane are identical, the end product in both cases being 2,5-hexanedione, which is considered to be the agent responsible for their neurotoxic effects.

Excretion

Both the quantity of ketones inhaled and the quantity excreted unchanged with the expired air depend on the volatility of the compound. The metabolites are excreted in the urine.

Assessment of exposure

Environmental assessment

Exposure to vapour may be assessed by air sampling and analysis in the breathing zone or by personal air samplers. However, the risk of skin absorption is not readily assessed.

Biological assessment

There are no reliable routine methods for the biological monitoring of exposure. The metabolic end-products of methyl n-butyl ketone (MBK) and methyl ethyl ketone can be measured in the urine, or, the unchanged ketones can be measured in the expired air, but the analytical methods are rather complicated and the exact relationship between exposure level and the amount excreted is not well established.

Clinical effects

Acute poisoning

All ketones are moderate irritants of mucous membranes. High-level exposure to ketones results in central nervous system depression and prenarcotic symptoms, which may progress to narcosis.

Chronic poisoning

Prolonged exposure to MBK (and to mixtures of MBK with methyl ethyl ketone) may produce a toxic sensory-motor peripheral neuropathy similar to that caused by other industrial toxins (e.g., carbon disulfide, acrylamide, and *n*-hexane). Sensory and motor impairment starts with symmetrical distribution of lesions in the distal part of the lower extremities and tends to involve progressively the upper extremities and the more proximal segments of the extremities. Muscle wasting may also be present in severe cases. Symptoms include loss of tactile sense and sensitivity to pain and temperature. Motor involvement is revealed by muscle weakness and diminished or lost deep tendon reflexes. Electromyographic abnormalities and reduction in nerve conduction velocity are always detectable and mostly precede clinical manifestations.

Exposure–effect relationship

For most of the saturated ketones the air concentrations causing slight eye irritation within a few minutes vary widely—from tens to hundreds of mg/m^3 of air. However, unsaturated ketones (such as vinyl methyl ketone) are much more powerful irritants, inducing the same degree of irritation at concentrations as low as around 5 mg/m^3. An exposure–effect relationship for MBK has not been established with certainty. Polyneuropathies were observed in workers exposed to concentrations of about 40 mg/m^3, but other ketones were also present in much higher concentrations.

Prognosis

Peripheral neuropathy has a protracted course. Recovery is not complete in all cases and some sensory and motor dysfunctions may remain as permanent sequelae.

Differential diagnosis

Peripheral neuropathy due to MBK exposure must be distinguished from neuropathies of other origins. Evidence of occupational exposure to MBK is essential.

Susceptibility

Individuals with pre-existing peripheral nervous impairment, those suffering from chronic liver and kidney diseases, and those who have lost their sense of smell are more susceptible than others.

Health examinations

Preplacement examination

The preplacement examination should include a medical history and a physical examination, with special attention to the central and peripheral nervous systems.

Periodic examinations

In medical terms, the periodic examination is the same as the preplacement one. In exposure to ketones for which chronic neurotoxicity has been demonstrated, the frequency is usually once or twice a year, depending on the exposure level. For high-risk subjects, neurological examination should include electroneurographic and behavioural testing.

Case management

There is no specific treatment for peripheral neuropathy or acute poisoning due to ketones. General supportive measures and rehabilitation therapy are useful.

Control measures

Occupational exposure to ketones may be controlled by enclosing process systems and by providing adequate ventilation in workrooms. Skin contact should be avoided or prevented by the wearing of gloves and protective clothing. Where high levels of exposure are possible (in poorly ventilated workrooms, heating operations, processes involving direct handling of ketones, etc.) workers should be provided with efficient means of protection against inhalation and skin contact (respirators, gloves, etc.).

Exposure limits for MBK vary in different countries from 20 mg/m^3 to 400 mg/m^3, for acetone from 200 to 2400 mg/m^3, for methyl isobutyl ketone from 300 mg/m^3 to 410 mg/m^3, and for methyl ethyl ketone from 200 mg/m^3 to 590 mg/m^3.

CHAPTER 22

Diseases caused by asphyxiants: carbon monoxide, hydrogen cyanide and its toxic derivatives, and hydrogen sulfide

CARBON MONOXIDE

Properties of the causal agent

Carbon monoxide (CO) is a colourless, odourless, tasteless, combustible, and explosive gas; it is lighter than air.

Occurrence and uses

Carbon monoxide is produced whenever there is incomplete burning of organic material. The following can be the potential sources of carbon monoxide: petrol and diesel powered internal combustion engines, boilers and furnaces, blasting operations, and fires.

Carbon monoxide is used in only a few industrial processes: in metallurgy as a reducing agent and in the chemical synthesis of, for example, carbonyls of metals, phosgene, formic acid, and methanol. Carbon monoxide is a component of coal gas. Hazardous concentrations are most likely to accumulate in confined spaces.

Occupations involving exposure to carbon monoxide

Workers in the manufacture and distribution of gas (coal gas) made from solid fuel, garage mechanics, engine operators, traffic personnel, acetylene welders, boiler-room workers, chemical workers, fire fighters, miners, etc. are at greatest risk. Non-occupational exposure occurs through tobacco smoking.

Mechanism of action

Absorption

Carbon monoxide is absorbed exclusively through the lungs.

154

Distribution

In blood, carbon monoxide binds with haemoglobin to form carboxyhaemoglobin, and in tissues, it binds with other iron-containing substances such as myoglobin, cytochromes, cytochrome oxidase, and catalase.

Excretion

Excretion takes place only by exhalation. The average biological half-life of carbon monoxide is about 5 hours. An increase in the partial pressure of oxygen in the inhaled air (i.e., breathing of oxygen-enriched air) reduces the half-life considerably.

Assessment of exposure

Environmental assessment

Detection tubes are useful for checking hazardous concentrations before entering contaminated areas. For area samples, several analytical methods may be used (e.g., infrared absorption and gas chromatography). Direct-reading instruments may also be used; these instruments provide continuous readings of peak and average concentrations.

Biological assessment

There are two biological methods of determining exposure: (*a*) by measuring the carboxyhaemoglobin concentration in blood; and (*b*) by measuring the carbon monoxide concentration in the expired air. Since carbon monoxide also occurs naturally in the body (as a product of haeme breakdown), so does carboxyhaemoglobin. The normal level of carboxyhaemoglobin in blood is up to 0.5 g/100 g haemoglobin, but if any haemolytic disorders are present, it may be as high as 5 g/100 g. Moreover, cigarette smoking may raise the level of carboxyhaemoglobin by 10% or more. Exposure to methylene chloride may also increase carboxyhaemoglobin levels. Hence, the above factors should be taken into account in considering the results of biological assessment.

There is a close relationship between the carboxyhaemoglobin level in arterial blood and the carbon monoxide concentration in alveolar air. A concentration in blood of 10 g of carboxyhaemoglobin per 100 g haemoglobin corresponds roughly to 55 g of carbon monoxide/m^3 of alveolar air. The most suitable methods for blood analysis are spectrophotometry, use of the Conway diffusion cell, and infrared absorption spectroscopy. Expired air may also be analysed by detection tubes.

Clinical effects

Acute poisoning

Exposure to high concentrations of carbon monoxide causes acute poisoning. Typical initial signs and symptoms are headache, dizziness, drowsiness, nausea, and vomiting. Depending on the concentration of CO in the air, duration of exposure, and resulting carboxyhaemoglobin concentration in the blood, collapse, coma, and death may occur. In individuals with arteriosclerosis, local ischaemic damage may occur in tissues where the blood supply is already reduced. The central nervous system and the heart muscle are the organs most sensitive to carbon monoxide poisoning.

Chronic poisoning

Experts appear to be divided on the issue of health impairment due to long-term exposure to concentrations of carbon monoxide insufficient to cause acute poisoning. While some believe that such exposure causes adverse effects others deny it. Those who believe in the occurrence of chronic poisoning, attribute the following symptoms to long-term carbon monoxide exposure: headache, memory defects, falling work output, sleep disturbances, vertigo, emotional lability, signs of central and peripheral nervous system impairment (encephalopathy, neuropathy) autonomic nervous system disorders (particularly impairment of its regulatory function over the cardiovascular system), and increased concentrations of serum cholesterol, lipoproteins, and glucose. It should be pointed out here that chronic poisoning should be distinguished from the effects of repeated episodes of slight acute poisoning.

Exposure–effect relationship

In acute poisoning, the amount of carboxyhaemoglobin formed depends on the concentration and duration of exposure to carbon monoxide and the intensity of lung ventilation (effect of heavy work). The first clinical signs and symptoms may appear at carboxyhaemoglobin levels of 15–20 g/100 g haemoglobin. Loss of consciousness occurs at a level of about 50 g/100 g.

Prognosis

Severe acute carbon monoxide poisoning may permanently damage the brain and heart muscle with residual local symptoms and signs. In less severe cases the prognosis is excellent.

Differential diagnosis

In acute poisoning, exclude other causes (neurological, metabolic) of impaired consciousness, and ascertain the presence of carbon monoxide in the blood or expired air. If chronic poisoning is suspected, neurological and cardiovascular diseases of other etiology should be excluded. A work history with evidence of elevated concentrations of carbon monoxide in breath and carboxyhaemoglobin in the blood and of repeated (slight) acute poisoning are important for the diagnosis of chronic poisoning.

Susceptibility

Any condition that impairs oxygen supply to vital organs (heart, brain, kidneys, anaemia) is likely to increase susceptibility.

Health examinations

Preplacement examination

The preplacement examination should include a medical history and a physical examination, with special attention to the cardiovascular and central nervous systems.

Periodic examinations

In medical terms, the periodic examination is the same as the preplacement one, and it is usually carried out at 1–2 year intervals.

Case management

In acute poisoning, immediately remove the patient from further exposure to carbon monoxide and administer oxygen until the carboxy-haemoglobin concentration in blood falls below 5 g/100 g haemoglobin. In some cases it may be necessary to give mouth-to-mouth respiration and an extrathoracic heart massage. Further treatment should be symptomatic. Patients with after-effects of acute poisoning should not be further employed in occupations involving exposure to carbon monoxide.

Control measures

Technical control measures should be applied to reduce carbon monoxide concentrations in the air and the possibility of its accidental escape. Continuous assessment of air concentrations is important.

Personal protective devices (clean air ventilation hood or apparatus with closed circuit of air in emergency situations) should be used whenever necessary. The recommended limits for carboxyhaemoglobin levels in blood for healthy and susceptible individuals are 5 g/100 g and 2.5 g/100 g haemoglobin, respectively.

Exposure limits (time-weighted average) in different countries vary from 20 mg/m³ to 55 mg/m³. Some countries have special regulations concerning short-term exposures (i.e., exposures lasting tens of minutes).

HYDROGEN CYANIDE AND ITS TOXIC DERIVATIVES

Properties of the causal agents

Hydrogen cyanide (HCN) is a colourless liquid with a typical odour of bitter almonds; it boils at 26 °C (at ambient temperatures, it may exist both as a liquid and as a gas). Its salts (potassium cyanide, sodium cyanide, etc.) are solids; they decompose easily on contact even with weak acids and release hydrogen cyanide. Acrylonitrile ($CH_2 = CHCN$) is a colourless, mobile liquid with a faint odour.

Uses

Hydrogen cyanide is used as a rodenticide, insecticide fumigant, and as a chemical intermediate in the manufacture of monomers (acrylonitrile, toluene diisocyanates). It is also used in the production of synthetic fibres or plastics, and cyanide salts are used in the extraction of gold and silver, electroplating, hardening of metals, manufacture of mirrors, photography, etc. Acrylonitrile is used in the manufacture of plastics.

Occupations involving exposure to hydrogen cyanide and its toxic derivatives

Fumigant workers, organic chemical synthesizers, electroplaters, gold and silver extractors, steel workers, and workers in the production of plastics (particularly acrylonitrile-styrene) are at greatest risk of exposure.

Mechanism of action

Absorption

Vapours of hydrogen cyanide and its compounds are absorbed through the lungs. A limited amount of skin absorption of the vapours is also possible. Liquids are easily absorbed through intact skin upon direct contact.

Biotransformation

Hydrogen cyanide has a strong affinity for trivalent iron and binds firmly to tissue enzymes containing it (cytochrome oxidases). The biotransformation of hydrogen cyanide and its salts is effected by reaction with proteins containing the SH-group (e.g., glutathion). As a result, thiocyanates (rhodanides) are formed. In the case of acrylonitrile, the molecule splits in the body and releases the cyanide group. Cyanides themselves are not toxic unless converted into hydrogen cyanide (e.g., by gastric juice which contains hydrochloric acid).

Excretion

Thiocyanates are excreted in the urine and faeces. Non-metabolized hydrogen cyanide is also excreted through breath. The biological half-life of hydrogen cyanide is between 20 and 60 min.

Assessment of exposure

Environmental assessment

Detector tubes may be used to measure air pollution levels in case of emergencies. Time-weighted average concentrations and peak values should be determined, preferably by personal sampling.

Biological assessment

The determination of the CN^- ion in blood or tissues is of significance only in acute poisoning. In occupational exposure to cyanides, the concentration of thiocyanates in the urine may be elevated, but the same is also true in smokers (tobacco smoke contains thiocyanates). In blood plasma of subjects not exposed occupationally, thiocyanates are present in concentrations up to 107 µg/litre; in the urine of non-smokers, thiocyanate concentrations reach up to 67 µg/litre and, in smokers, up to 174 µg/litre.

Clinical effects

Hydrogen cyanide, its salts and acrylonitrile are weak irritants to the eyes and mucous membranes. Of major importance in the systemic poisoning by hydrogen cyanide is the inhibition of several metabolic enzyme systems, particularly cytochrome oxidase, the enzyme involved in the ultimate transfer of electrons to molecular oxygen. Since cytochrome oxidase is present in all cells, all aerobic cellular respiration is impaired, and anoxia develops in spite of normal quantities of oxygen in the blood.

Acute effects

Initial symptoms of acute hydrogen cyanide poisoning include weakness, headache, confusion, and, occasionally, nausea and vomiting. In severe cases, coma, convulsions, and death due to respiratory arrest may occur.

Chronic effects

It is claimed that long-term exposure to hydrogen cyanide, cyanide derivatives and acrylonitrile induce nonspecific symptoms that affect several body systems. However, the occurrence of chronic cyanide poisoning is not universally accepted. The following conditions are allegedly caused by chronic exposure to hydrogen cyanide and its derivatives: neurasthenia with autonomic nervous system involvement, psychic alterations, precordial pains, breathlessness on exertion, bradycardia, arterial hypotonia, polycythaemia, dyspepsia, hepatic impairment, and thyroidal hypofunction. Allergic dermatoses due to skin contact with certain cyanides have been observed.

Exposure–effect relationship

Lethal concentrations for humans have been assessed at about: $300 \, mg/m^3$ for 6–8 min exposure; $200 \, mg/m^3$ for 10 min; and $150 \, mg/m^3$ for 30 min. No exposure–effect relationship for chronic poisoning has been established.

Prognosis

The prognosis of acute hydrogen cyanide poisoning depends on the extent and duration of tissue hypoxia. In severe poisoning, incapacitating encephalopathy, paresis, myocardial damage, etc., may persist. Prognosis of mild poisoning is excellent.

Differential diagnosis

In acute poisoning, exclude other causes of comatose states (nervous, cardiovascular, metabolic disorder and other poisonings). Evidence of high-level exposure (work history, biological assessment) must be present. If chronic poisoning with hydrogen cyanide is suspected, other etiologies must be excluded by a careful examination.

Susceptibility

Persons with affections of the organs that are targets for hydrogen cyanide poisoning (brain, heart muscle) are likely to be more susceptible than others.

Health examinations

Preplacement examination

The preplacement examination should include a medical history and a physical examination, with special attention to the nervous and cardiovascular systems.

Periodic examination

In medical terms, the periodic examination is the same as the preplacement one. It is usually carried out once every year.

Case management

Acute hydrogen cyanide poisoning can be treated very efficiently. The patient should be immediately removed from further exposure, and contaminated skin should be washed with warm water and soap. With as little delay as possible, amyl nitrite should be administered by inhalation in order to form methaemoglobin which binds firmly with free cyanide ions to form cyanmethaemoglobin. A more effective treatment is sodium nitrite given intravenously. Thereafter, sodium thiosulfate is given intravenously to increase the rate of conversion of cyanide to thiocyanate. Recently, hydroxocobalamin has been shown to be even more effective than the classical treatments described above. Nonspecific supportive therapy (artificial breathing, etc.) may also be necessary. First-aid kits with antidotes should be kept handy wherever there is a risk of cyanide poisoning.

Control measures

Exposure should be restricted by technical control measures. Personal protective devices may be necessary. Instruments for the automatic determination and warning of dangerous concentrations may be useful.

Exposure limits for hydrogen cyanide in different countries vary between $0.3 \mu g/m^3$ and $11 \mu g/m^3$; for acrylonitrile the range is $0.5-45 \mu g/m^3$.

HYDROGEN SULFIDE

Properties of the causal agent

Hydrogen sulfide (H_2S) is a flammable colourless gas with a typical rotten-egg odour. It is heavier than air.

Occurrence and uses

In nature, hydrogen sulfide occurs in volcanic gases and in damp areas where sulfur-containing organic material is decomposing by bacterial action. In industrial operations, it may be formed whenever elemental sulfur or some sulfur-containing compound comes into contact with organic materials at high temperatures. Hydrogen sulfide also occurs as an undesirable by-product in many industries. These include: petrochemical industries; coke plants; factories producing viscose rayon, cellophane, barium salts, and sulfur-containing dyes and pigments; lithography and photogravure workshops; beet sugar plants; leather tanneries; and sewage treatment plants.

Hydrogen sulfide is used as a chemical intermediate in the synthesis of inorganic sulfides, sulfuric acid, and organic sulfur compounds.

Occupations involving exposure to hydrogen sulfide

Sewage treatment plant workers, miners, metallurgists, silo workers, sugar beet processers, tannery workers, viscose rayon and cellophane workers, chemical plant workers (manufacturing of sulfuric acids, barium salts, etc.) are at greatest risk of exposure.

Mechanism of action

Absorption

In occupational exposure, absorption takes place by inhalation only.

Biotransformation

Hydrogen sulfide undergoes rapid oxidation to sulfates. It acts as an inhibitor of cytochrome oxidase (Warburg's respiratory enzyme).

Excretion

Only a small proportion (less than 10%) of the amount absorbed is excreted unchanged in expired air. The metabolites of hydrogen sulfide (sulfates, thiosulfates) are excreted in the urine.

Assessment of exposure

Environmental assessment

Detection tubes may be used to measure pollution levels in areas where hazardous concentrations are likely to occur. For quantitative determination of air concentrations, both the methylene blue colorimetric method and gas-chromatography are recommended. Note that the latter permits personal sampling.

Biological assessment

There are no methods of biological assessment.

Clinical effects

Acute effects

Hydrogen sulfide has a direct irritant action on the eyes, which sometimes leads to keratoconjunctivitis. It is also an irritant of the respiratory tract, and may cause bronchitis or even pulmonary oedema. High concentrations have paralysing effects on the olfactory apparatus and the odour of the gas is no longer perceived. Symptoms of acute poisonings include: irritation of the eyes and airways, headache, vertigo, giddiness, and retrosternal pain. In severe poisoning, coma, convulsions, and death may occur, sometimes within a few seconds.

Chronic poisoning

Nonspecific symptoms and disorders such as impaired sleep, headache, vertigo, poor concentration, lability of mood, hyperhydrosis, autonomic nervous system impairment, chronic bronchitis, and dyspepsia are accepted by some authorities as resulting from long-term exposure to concentrations of hydrogen sulfide lower than those causing acute poisoning. Others do not accept the existence of chronic poisoning.

Exposure–effect relationship

The threshold for identifying hydrogen sulfide by smell is about $0.012-0.03\,\mu g/m^3$ air. At $7-11\,\mu g/m^3$ the odour is intolerable, even by those exposed to it regularly. The inhalation of air containing $1500\,\mu g/m^3$ can cause coma after a single breath and death rapidly ensues. Prolonged exposure to $375\,\mu g/m^3$ causes pulmonary oedema, and exposure to $75\,\mu g/m^3$ causes keratoconjunctivitis and bronchitis.

Prognosis

Severe acute poisoning with coma may result in permanent damage to the brain or heart, whereas the prognosis of mild poisoning is favourable.

Differential diagnosis

Exclude other causes of impaired consciousness (neurological, cardiovascular, metabolic) and prove high-level exposure to hydrogen sulfide (on the basis of work history, evidence of high concentrations in the air). In the case of keratoconjunctivitis or acute respiratory disease, evidence of high-level exposure alone may be sufficient.

Susceptibility

Diseases causing impaired supply of oxygen to vital organs (arteriosclerosis of the brain or of coronary arteries, anaemia, chronic respiratory diseases, and keratoconjunctivitis) may all increase susceptibility.

Health examinations

Preplacement examination

The preplacement examination should include a medical history and a physical examination, with special attention to the eyes and the nervous, cardiovascular and respiratory systems. Optionally, basic lung function tests (FVC, $FEV_{1.0}$) may be carried out.

Periodic examinations

In medical terms the periodic examination is the same as the preplacement one, and is carried out usually at least once a year.

Case management

In acute poisoning, immediately remove the patient from exposure and start symptomatic treatment. Artificial respiration may be necessary.

Control measures

Air concentrations of hydrogen sulfide should be limited by technical control measures (enclosed systems, ventilation). Respiratory protection (respirators or closed-circuit device) may be necessary.

Exposure limits for hydrogen sulfide in the air of workplaces in different countries range between $10\,\mu g/m^3$ and $15\,\mu g/m^3$.

CHAPTER 23

Hearing impairment caused by noise

Properties of the causal agent

Noise is generally defined as any unwanted sound. Sound is sensation produced in the ear by the vibrations of the air or other media. Sound can also be perceived by direct contact with vibrating objects. The human ear is capable of perceiving sound in the range of 16–20 000 Hz. A narrow-band noise has most of the energy confined to a narrow range of frequencies, and a pure tone (e.g., that produced by a tuning-fork) consists of a sound of a single, very constant frequency. In the case of wide-band noise, acoustical energy is distributed over a large range of frequencies.

The harmfulness of noise is related to several factors:

Intensity. The sound intensity perceived by the ear is directly proportional to the logarithm of the square of the acoustic pressure produced by vibrations in the audible range. Accordingly, the sound pressure level is measured on a logarithmic scale in decibels (dB).

Frequency. The sound frequencies audible to the human ear lie between 16 Hz and 20 000 Hz. The frequencies comprising speech are in the range of 250–4000 Hz. High frequency sounds are the more dangerous.

Duration. The adverse effect of noise is proportional to the duration of exposure, and appears to be related to the total amount of energy reaching the inner ear. Thus, it is desirable to measure all the elements of the acoustic environment (despite the difficulty of doing so); recording and integrating noise-meters are used for this purpose.

Nature. This refers to the distribution of the sound energy over time (stable, fluctuating, intermittent). Impulsive noise (one or more bursts of sound energy of less than 1 second's duration) is particularly harmful.

Occupations involving exposure to noise

In industry, increased mechanization results in increased noise levels. The occupations that carry a particularly high risk of hearing loss include: mining, tunnelling, quarrying (detonations, drilling), heavy engineering (iron casting, forging presses, etc.), operation of machinery driven by powerful combustion engines (trucks, construction vehicles etc.), operation of textile machines, and testing of jet engines.

Mechanism of action and types of hearing loss

Under experimental conditions, very loud sound in the audible range causes irreversible lesions of the cochlea. The early changes affect the cells at the base of the cochlea.

Hearing loss can be either temporary or permanent. Noise-induced temporary threshold shift (NITTS, or auditory fatigue) is a temporary loss of hearing acuity experienced after a relatively short exposure to excessive noise. Hearing recovers fairly rapidly after the cessation of the noise. Noise-induced permanent threshold shift (NIPTS) is an irreversible loss of hearing that is caused by prolonged exposure to noise. Noise-induced threshold shift is the quantity of hearing loss attributable to noise alone (after values for presbyacusis have been subtracted). Hearing impairment is generally referred to as the hearing level at which individuals experience difficulty in leading a normal life, usually in understanding speech.

Assessment of exposure

Environmental assessment

Industrial noise measurement equipment incorporates sound filters of different types (A, B, C), the measurements recorded by different filters being expressed as dB(A), dB(B), dB(C), respectively. Noise is most frequently measured in dB(A). However, since noise measurements with these instruments do not register impulsive noise, it is common to add 10 dB to the measured value when the impulsive type of noise is present.

Use is also made of dosimetric techniques to record the sound energy build-up over a period of time. To measure an average sound level the meter averaging time is extended to equal the period of interest (commonly 8 hours). This gives the equivalent continuous sound pressure level (L_{eq}).

Biological assessment

Hearing impairment has been defined as an arithmetic average of 26–30 dB or more of hearing loss at defined frequencies (500, 1000, 2000, 4000 Hz), which vary from country to country. Audiometric monitoring of exposed workers may be at variance with the theoretical risk as appraised by noise measurement. This discrepancy is explained by the difficulty of making an allowance for the real amount of sound energy reaching the ear, owing to the presence of impulsive noises.

Clinical effects

The characteristics of hearing loss caused by occupational noise exposure are as follows:

—There is inner ear hearing loss, with superpositioning of aerial and bone conduction and recruitment.

—The hearing loss is bilateral and more or less symmetrical.

—The loss commences at a frequency of 4000 Hz. At this stage there is a characteristic V-shaped notch in the audiogram. This condition is latent (the only difficulty is in hearing whispers), and its identification requires systematic detection procedures. After a further period of exposure, the hearing loss deteriorates and extends to a broader range of frequencies, and the impairment then becomes apparent. If further exposure is not stopped, the loss worsens and may reach near deafness.

—Once deafness occurs, it is permanent and stable even after the acoustic hazard has been removed.

Sometimes, there may be variations in the clinical picture: for example, the loss may be predominantly unilateral. This may be due to the position of the head during work, especially when the noise is highly pulsating in nature.

Acute apoplexy may be encountered in workers exposed to loud noise during explosions or other accidents at work. Some forms of noise-induced apoplexy begin at low frequencies (less than 500 Hz). The workers usually affected by these conditions include test-bed workers and workers employed on the repair of jet engines. In these cases deafness is severe and the condition progresses rapidly.

Exposure–effect relationship

It is now accepted that the risk of hearing damage is negligible at noise levels of $\leqslant$ 75 dB(A) L_{eq} for a daily exposure of 8 hours. Even at exposure levels of up to 80 dB(A), there is no detectable increase in the percentage of subjects with hearing impairment. At 85 dB(A), however, there is a probability that after 5 years of work, 1% of workers will exhibit some (usually minor) hearing loss; after 10 years of work, 3% of workers are likely to show hearing loss, and after 15 years, 5% of them will do so. At a noise level of 90 dB(A), the respective percentages are 4%, 10%, and 14%, and at 95 dB(A), the percentages are 7%, 17%, and 24%, respectively.

Prognosis

In general, hearing impairment caused by noise develops over many years of exposure. The rate of deterioration depends on the level, the impulsive component, and the duration of the exposure, and also on individual sensitivity, the nature of which remains unknown. Some other pathological conditions contribute to hearing impairment, such as intoxication, injury, and, from the age of 55 years onwards, presbyacusis. The influence of disease of the middle ear on susceptibility to noise is disputed, with the exception of the fairly late stage of labyrinthitis. Hearing impairment may accompany changes in the vascular and nervous systems, including asthenia and neurotic states.

Differential diagnosis

Exclude damage to the auditory nerve (due to infection or poisoning) otosclerosis, and middle ear disease resulting from chronic otitis.

Susceptibility

It has been postulated that persons with a history of meningitis, treatment with an ototoxic drug, a familial tendency towards early deafness, diabetes, or arterial hypertension may be more susceptible to hearing loss from exposure to noise. The effect of otitis and middle ear infections on susceptibility is uncertain. However, if any pathological condition of the ear is detected in a worker exposed to noise, precautions are advisable.

Tests of auditory fatigue have been suggested for the detection of individual susceptibility to noise. In such tests the auditory threshold is first measured at a frequency of 4000 Hz and then the ear is exposed to sound of a known high intensity for a given time (e.g., sound frequency of 2000 Hz, 80 dB, for eight minutes). Once again the auditory threshold is measured at 4000 Hz and the difference in auditory threshold before and after exposure represents auditory fatigue. However, no exact correlation has been established between the risk of deafness and auditory threshold shift.

Health examinations

Preplacement examination

The preplacement examination should include a medical history and a physical examination, with special attention to hearing acuity. Audiometric screening is also recommended.

Periodic examination

In medical terms, the periodic examination is the same as the preplacement one. It should be carried out once every year, and should include annual audiometric screening by pure-tone audiometry. This screening can be carried out in the factory, provided that a suitable low-noise-level cabin is available. Otherwise it should be done in a specially equipped room or in an audiometric van.

Case management

Transfer the patient away from noisy work in order to stop further deterioration.

Control measures

The essential measure is the reduction of sound levels, by technical means, either as a corrective measure (sound-absorbing, antireflection panels, baffle-plating, hooding, etc.) or, preferably, by designing less noisy machinery.

Individual protection entails education and persuasion of workers to use protective gear. Plastic ear-plugs, which are sometimes poorly tolerated, and wax-impregnated disposable plugs reduce noise levels by between 8 dB and 30 dB. Muff-type ear defenders and headphones are more effective (20–40 dB reduction). Although they are uncomfortable to wear, they are essential when there is brief exposure to very high sound levels (e.g., the noise levels experienced by airport personnel during the guiding of landings).

There are many national and international standards that define the danger thresholds for the ear as a function of the level of sound intensity and frequency. As a general rule, the threshold for adverse effects for an 8-hour daily exposure is set at 85 dB at a frequency of 1000 Hz. Tables showing similar threshold values for other frequencies and duration of exposure during the work-shift are available.

CHAPTER 24

Diseases caused by vibration

Properties of the causal agent

The main characteristics of vibration are frequency (in Hz) and intensity (measured as amplitude, velocity, or acceleration).

Vibration may be transmitted to the entire body (whole-body vibration) or only to the arm holding a vibrating tool or device (localized vibration). Only the effects of localized vibration are discussed in this chapter.

Occurrence and uses

Vibrating tools are widely used in metal, shipbuilding, and automotive industries as well as in mining, forestry, and construction work. The most common vibrating tools are: pneumatic drills, vibratory chisels, grinding appliances, motor saws, polishing machines, and pneumatic hammers. These tools produce mechanical vibrations of different physical characteristics, which have different adverse effects.

Occupations involving exposure to vibrations

Operators of pneumatic drills, vibratory chisels, chain-saws, grinders, riveters, etc. are at greatest risk of exposure.

Mechanism of action

Vibration is measured by determining the quantity of mechanical energy transmitted per surface unit during a certain period of time; this mechanical energy is a function of the frequency and intensity of the oscillating movement producing the vibration. The quantity of absorbed energy is a function of the frequency, intensity, and duration of vibration. The transmission and dissipation of vibratory energy in man depends on the intensity of the vibration, the direction of action of the vibration, body posture, muscular tension, the physical properties of the body, and anthropometric features.

Assessment of exposure

The evaluation of exposure is a difficult and complex problem. The methods and range of measurements and their interpretation have so far not been unified. The International Organization for Standardization is developing principles for the measurement and evaluation of exposure to vibration transmitted to the hand.[1]

Clinical effects

The effects of vibration on the hands are various nonspecific symptoms defined collectively as the vibration syndrome. The major disturbances are those of the vascular system, peripheral nerves, and the skeletomuscular system.

Angioneurosis of the fingers

Raynaud's phenomenon (white fingers) is the most frequent vibration-induced syndrome in the cooler regions of the world.

The first nonspecific symptoms are acroparaesthesias of the hands or a feeling of numbness in the fingers during work or shortly afterwards. At this stage, apart from disturbed vibration sensitivity, no other objective changes are found. In the next phase, sporadic paroxysmal paleness of some finger tips is observed. The paroxysm is caused by local spasm of the arterioles and capillaries and is triggered by exposure to local or general cold. It usually occurs in cold weather and is fully reversible in 15–30 min after warming of hands. During the paroxysm, tactile pain sensitivity is much diminished. This phase of the disease poses the greatest diagnostic difficulties, since the reported ailment cannot always be confirmed by examination in the physician's consulting room. The observation of an attack directly at the workplace facilitates its diagnosis.

The more advanced stage of the disease is characterized by paroxysmal pallor, which affects not only the tips but spreads over most of the fingers, but rarely affects the thumbs. The paroxysm is provoked even by slight cold, though it may appear at ambient temperatures as well. In the most advanced stages, angiospasm is replaced by paresis of small vessel walls, resulting in acrocyanosis. The predominant symptoms are numbness of the hands, impairment of finger dexterity, and disturbed sensitivity. Local changes in tone may also develop. In contrast to obliterating endarteritis, necrosis is extremely rare.

The most common diagnostic test used is the induction of the finger paroxysm by cold water. Both hands and forearms (up to the elbows)

[1] International Organization for Standardization. *Principles for the measurement and evaluation of human exposure to vibration transmitted to the hand.* Geneva, ISO, 1976 (ISO/DIS 5349).

are kept immersed for 10 min in water cooled with ice-cubes. (Some physicians increase the general coolness by putting a wet towel on the subject's shoulders.) It should be pointed out that this method induces finger paroxysm less frequently than do vibrations in a real work situation.

Sometimes only delayed return of blood into the capillaries can be demonstrated: the finger tip above the nail should be briefly compressed and the time taken by the blood to return to the anoxaemic spot registered.

Laboratory examination methods applicable in preventive examinations include finger plethysmography (impairment of the pulse wave by cold), capillary microscopy, and skin temperature measurement (by contact thermometer or thermography). There may be a lower initial skin temperature or delay in the re-establishment of normal finger temperature after the cold-water test.

Bone, joint, and muscular disorders

Osteoarticular pathology is mostly localized to the carpal bones (especially lunate and navicular), radioulnar joints, and elbow joints. There are usually only minor subjective symptoms. At an advanced stage, however, functional impairment may be significant.

The most typical X-ray changes are arthrosis of the carpal, radioulnar, and elbow joints and pseudocysts (particularly in the carpal bones, which may also show other atrophic changes, such as thickened and rarified trabeculae).

In advanced cases, even fragmentation of the articular surface, free joint bodies, or chronic fractures or breakages of bone fragments may occur. Aseptic necrosis of the lunate bone is known under various terms (e.g., osteomalacia of traumatic origin, Kienböck's disease, lunatomalacia).

The muscles or tendons surrounding the joints are usually also involved; the subjective symptoms (pain) caused by these affections often precede demonstrable X-ray changes.

Neuropathy

Damage to the nerves due to vibrations includes disturbances of the peripheral autonomic innervation (in angioneurosis). Effects on the peripheral nerves (ulnar, median, radial) are claimed by some authors. Other specialists consider nerve injury as mostly secondary to either repeated ischaemia (in angioneurosis) or to an additional factor, most frequently, compressive neuropathy (e.g., osteoarticular changes in the neighbourhood of the nerve stem). Affection of sensory fibres causes paresthesia or diminished sensitivity of motor fibres, impaired dexterity, and later, atrophy. The measurement of nerve conduction velocity is the examination of choice.

A mixed form combines disturbances of muscles, tendons, bones, vessels and peripheral nerves.

Exposure–effect relationship

The frequencies that commonly cause adverse health effects are in the range of 30–1000 Hz (the amplitude being about 100 µm), although vibrations of over 150 Hz cause symptoms infrequently. While hammer-type tools produce vibrations of mostly 30–50 Hz, oscillatory and rotary tools sometimes produce vibrations of up to 1000 Hz.

The disturbances induced by vibration may appear after different lengths of time following the onset of exposure. Angioneurosis usually appears after several years of exposure, but sometimes it develops within several months of heavy exposure. Skeletal changes normally arise not earlier than after 10 years or more of exposure.

Prognosis

The interruption of exposure at the early (angiospastic) stage may allow the symptoms to regress. Advanced vascular and nervous disturbances are rarely fully reversible. The osseoarticular pathologies are irreversible, but the impairment of hand and arm movements occurs only in advanced stages.

Differential diagnosis

Exclude other disorders of peripheral blood vessels such as secondary Raynaud's phenomenon and Raynaud's disease, scleroderma, thromboangiitis obliterans, arteriosclerosis obliterans, cryoglobulinaemia, and frostbite. Also exclude disorders of peripheral nerves and neuropathies of other origin, particularly the compressive ones.

In cases involving disorders of muscles, bones, and joints, exclude rheumatoid arthritis, osteoarthritis deformans, sequelae of trauma, and fractures.

Susceptibility

Persons under 20 years of age are particularly vulnerable to the effects of vibration. Adverse effects of vibration are enhanced by the presence of autonomic dysfunction, diseases of peripheral vessels and nerves, previous frostbite of the hands, and trauma of the upper limbs.

Health examination

Preplacement examination

The preplacement examination should include a medical history and a physical examination, with special attention to the peripheral circulation and the nervous and locomotor systems.

Periodic examination

In medical terms, the periodic examination is the same as the preplacement one. It is usually carried out once a year, but if exposure limits are considerably exceeded or if workers rapidly progress to advanced stages of vibration-related diseases, more frequent examinations may be necessary. Since bone changes take several years to appear, an X-ray examination should be done at 5-year intervals. In advanced cases, the interval should be 2–3 years.

Case management

When adverse effects of vibration become apparent in a worker, he should be removed from further exposure. There is no specific treatment, but in cases of advanced vascular changes the use of vasodilators and physiotherapeutic and balneotherapeutic procedures is recommended.

Control measures

The hazardous effects of occupational exposure to vibration may be best prevented by improving the design of the vibrating tools and by using protective "anti-vibration" gloves. The proper maintenance of instruments is also important. The risk may also be decreased by shortening the time of exposure.

Properly conducted preplacement and periodic examinations facilitate the early recognition of those particularly vulnerable and help in reducing the extent of the problem.

The International Organization for Standardization has recommended provisional exposure limits for hand-transmitted vibration in the frequency range of 8–1000 Hz.[1] The limits are specified in terms of one-third octave band and octave band, vibration acceleration or velocity, daily exposure time, intermittency of exposure, and direction of vibration relative to the hand.

[1] See footnote on page 171.

CHAPTER 25

Diseases caused by compressed air

Properties of the causal agent

Compressed air is air at pressures higher than that at sea level (normal atmospheric pressure).

Uses

Caissons filled with compressed air are used for the underwater construction and repair of tunnels and bridge piers. For most practical purposes compressed air in caissons is limited to a maximum pressure of about 330 kPa. At pressures greater than this commercial tunnelling or caisson work becomes economically prohibitive because the decompression time becomes too long.

Occupations involving exposure to compressed air

Workers in compressed air tunnelling and caisson operations and divers are at greatest risk.

Mechanism of action

Compressed air may cause either mechanical effects (barotrauma) or physiological effects (due to the elevated partial pressure of its component gases). Whereas the former are caused by a difference in pressure on the two sides of the tympanic membrane, the major effect of the latter (decompression sickness) is due to the formation of nitrogen bubbles in the blood. Under normal atmospheric pressure, about 12 ml of nitrogen are dissolved in 1 litre of blood. At a pressure of 196 kPa, the nitrogen concentration in blood is about 22 ml/litre, and at 390 kPa the concentration is about 39 ml/litre. If decompression to atmospheric pressure is excessively rapid, the nitrogen dissolved in the blood forms bubbles in the blood and tissues, causing circulatory impairment and local tissue damage.

Assessment of exposure

Exposure depends on three factors: (*a*) pressure of compressed air; (*b*) the depth under water at which caissons are being used; and (*c*) duration of exposure.

Clinical effects

The adverse health effects of compressed air exposure include: middle-ear and sinus barotrauma, burst lung and cerebral air embolism, decompression sickness, oxygen toxicity (if oxygen is used during decompression), and osteonecrosis due to dysbarism.

Middle-ear and sinus barotrauma

This is the most common health problem experienced by compressed air workers. If the eustachian tube is blocked for any reason (e.g., due to upper respiratory tract infection), the air pressure in the middle ear cannot equalize with the air pressure surrounding the body and consequently, the ear-drum can become physically damaged or ruptured. Rupture of the round or oval window may also occur if the individual does a forceful Valsalva's manoeuvre in an effort to open the eustachian tube; the Valsalva's manoeuvre causes increased intracranial pressure to be transmitted to the endolymph and this forces the round or oval window into the middle-ear space where there is a relative vacuum. If the Valsalva's manoeuvre is not done, the tympanic membrane usually ruptures first. Symptoms include immediate tinnitus and deafness, and sometimes, disturbances of equilibrium and nystagmus.

During compression, the sinus cavities must be open otherwise there is severe pain. The frontal sinuses are the ones that are most commonly involved and also the ones that are most painful.

Burst lung with cerebral air embolism

During decompression, if there is an obstruction of the trachea or of a bronchiopulmonary segment and if the alveolar pressure rises by 10.8 kPa (80 mm Hg) above the intrapleural pressure, the lung may burst. Air embolism of the brain can be the most serious consequence of exposure to compressed air. However, in tunnelling work the slow decompression procedure used is extremely unlikely to cause burst lung. The symptoms of cerebral air embolism are hemiplegia, unconsciousness, and convulsions. Death may ensue within 1 or 2 minutes. Other complications include pneumomediastinum with subcutaneous emphysema, pneumopericardium, and pneumothorax (if the pleura ruptures).

Decompression sickness

Decompression sickness is of two types:

Type I decompression sickness. In this condition, there are no other symptoms except pain, which usually occurs in the extremities in muscles or tendons, commonly near a joint. About 90 % of all persons with decompression sickness report pain. In tunnel workers using compressed air caissons, pain in the lower extremities is most common.

Type II decompression sickness. This is a more serious condition. It includes spinal cord and brain injury, inner-ear disturbances, pulmonary embarrassment, and decompression sickness shock. Spinal cord dysfunction may cause numbness, paresthesia, or frank paralysis, commonly of the lower extremities; rarely, quadriplegia may result. The brain is usually spared in decompression sickness in tunnel workers. About 25 % of all cases have neurological complaints.

Vestibular decompression sickness ("staggers") is seen in about 5 % of cases, with severe true vertigo, nystagmus, nausea, and vomiting. Pulmonary embarrassment ("chokes") occurs in about 6 % of the cases, and is characterized by increasing difficulty in drawing a deep breath and paroxyms of choking cough. If left untreated, it will eventually lead to asphyxia.

Shock in decompression sickness can be severe enough to cause death. Pulmonary oedema is also a striking feature of shock; fortunately this is rare.

Dysbaric osteonecrosis (aseptic necrosis)

In the mid-1960s, degeneration of the hip and shoulder joints resulting from improper decompression was found in certain countries to afflict up to 20 % of compressed air tunnel workers and up to 35 % of other compressed air workers. With more modern decompression schedules, the disease has been reduced dramatically, but after long exposure to high pressures it still occurs. Shaft lesions of distal femur and proximal tibia are the mildest form of this disorder and produce no symptoms. With more severe exposure, the hips and shoulders are affected, but not other joints. The earliest radiographic signs of the disease appear at 3–4 months after exposure to improper decompression; a single episode of improper decompression may precipitate the ultimate destruction of one or more joints.

Exposure–effect relationship

Sinus pains appear at a very low difference of pressure. The eardrum ruptures at a pressure difference of about 49 kPa, but the lung may rupture at a pressure difference of only about 10.8 kPa.

In spite of all the currently employed safety procedures decompression sickness is still common in compressed air tunnel workers. The incidence rates of compressed-air-related disorders vary between 1 %

and 26% for each workshift. The exposure–effect relationship is complicated. The amount of nitrogen dissolved in the blood and tissues depends on the degree and duration of exposure to pressure and on the amount of body fat in which the nitrogen is dissolved. The amount of nitrogen bubbles formed depends on the quantity of nitrogen dissolved in the blood and on the rapidity of decompression (to ground-level pressure) from elevated air pressure. Dysbaric osteonecrosis does not usually appear at pressures less than 113 kPa.

Prognosis

Acute symptoms and signs are usually fully reversible if the patient undergoes rapid treatment by recompression. However, permanent damage or death may also occur. The prognosis of dysbaric osteonecrosis is uncertain.

Differential diagnosis

Recompression usually relieves the symptoms and signs of acute decompression sickness. If there is no relief, other causes of acute cardiovascular or nervous system impairment should be sought. In cases of dysbaric osteonecrosis, osteoarthritis of other origin should be excluded.

Susceptibility

Obstruction of air passages or of the external or internal ear, gross obesity, age, and illness, increase susceptibility.

Health examinations

Preplacement examination

The preplacement examination should include a medical history and a physical examination, with special attention to the respiratory system (air passages, lungs), ears and hearing, and nervous and locomotor systems. X-rays of the shoulders, hips, and knees should be taken, with special views for osteonecrosis.

Periodic examinations

In medical terms, the periodic examination is the same as the preplacement one. In the case of workers who work at pressures in excess of 106 kPa, X-rays should be taken at yearly intervals.

Case management

Patients with round or oval window rupture require bed rest, and if symptoms do not clear within 48 hours, the patient should be examined by a specialist. Pneumothorax may require surgical treatment. In case of air embolism in the brain, the only treatment is immediate recompression to 490 kPa in a recompression or hyperbaric chamber. In decompression sickness, recompression in a hyperbaric chamber (to allow nitrogen bubbles to disappear) followed by careful decompression is the only definitive therapy. In the case of shock, intravenous fluid should be administered in order to maintain blood volume.

When oxygen is used for decompression, the possibility of oxygen toxicity should be kept in mind. Oxygen under pressure is clinically toxic to the lungs and central nervous system. Six hours of continuous breathing of 100% oxygen at pressures up to 98 kPa will cause decreased vital capacity, chest pain, patchy atelectasis, and loss of surfactant. At pressures greater than 98 kPa, there are adverse effects on the central nervous system. After three hours of continuous breathing of 100% oxygen at 196 kPa, most individuals develop grand mal seizures.

Prevention

The only way of preventing decompression sickness is by careful adherence to the prescribed decompression work practices.

CHAPTER 26

Diseases caused by ionizing radiation

Properties of the causal agent

Ionizing radiation comprises those forms of radiation that, upon interaction with matter, give rise to particles of opposite electrical charges (ions). Ionizing radiation (both natural and artificial) is of two types: electromagnetic and corpuscular. The former is characterized by a frequency range of more than 3.0×10^{15} Hz (wavelength less than 1.0×10^{-17} m) and energy per photon range (eV) of more than 1.2×10^1 (X-rays, gamma-rays). Corpuscular radiation comprises alpha and beta particles, electrons, protons, deuterons, neutrons, etc.

Occurrence and uses

Ionizing radiation has always been a part of man's natural environment (cosmic rays, natural radioelements). Today, man-made ionizing radiation is widely used in industry, agriculture, medicine and scientific research. The sources of ionizing radiation are either high-energy electrical devices (X-ray machines or particle accelerators such as betatrons) or radionuclides (natural or artificial). Radionuclides are used either fully encapsulated (sealed sources) or as tracers added directly to the study systems (unsealed sources).

Occupations involving exposure to ionizing radiation

Persons at greatest risk of exposure to ionizing radiation include: uranium miners and mill workers, nuclear reactor and atomic energy plant workers, industrial radiographers (including those doing field work involving pipeline welding), certain health personnel (radiologists), workers employed in the production of radionuclides, scientists using radioactive material for research, and luminous dial painters.

Mechanism of action

The absorption of radiant energy by the tissues leads to adverse biological effects. The amount of radiant energy absorbed by the tissues depends on the wavelength of the radiation and the energy,

180

size, and charge of the particles. X-rays and gamma-rays of short wavelength and neutron particles travel a long distance in the air and penetrate deep into the tissues before being absorbed (having transferred their energy to the media they travel through). On the other hand, X-rays of long wavelength and alpha-particles travel only a few millimetres in the air, and are absorbed by thin layers of matter (tissues of less than a few millimetres' thickness). The unit of absorbed dose of radiation is the gray (Gy) (1 Gy = 1 J/kg = 100 rad).

Exposure to ionizing radiation occurs in two ways: externally and internally.

(1) *External exposure* to radiation occurs from sources localized outside the body. The effects of external exposure depend on the penetrating power of the radiation: it is mainly the outer integument that absorbs most of the radiation of a low penetrating power, whereas highly penetrating radiation reaches deep-seated tissues and organs.

(2) *Internal exposure* is caused by radioactive substances that have entered the body. Radioactive substances enter the body mainly by inhalation (radioactive dusts, vapours, or gases), although entry by ingestion (swallowing of contaminated food, water, etc.) and skin penetration (particularly through wounds in case of accidents) may also be significant. The mechanisms of absorption, distribution, bio-transformation, and excretion of radionuclides are the same as those of their non-radioactive counterparts. The only difference is in residence time, which, in the case of radioactive substances, depends on both metabolism and radioactive decay of the radionuclide.

Assessment of exposure

Environmental assessment

Geiger–Müller counters and scintillation counters are used for the detection of the presence of ionizing particles and the determination of the concentration of radioactive isotopes in the body, respectively. They are used also for the detection of radioactive contamination of surfaces or skin. If they are used for the measurement of the absorbed dose or of the rate of absorption, they must be calibrated for the particular type of radiation energy being measured.

Dosimeters used for measurement of ionizing radiation include: (*a*) ionizing chambers, film strips, or thermoluminescent devices. They are most suitable for personal monitoring of the doses received by the individuals who carry them on their suits in all work locations. Usually, pocket dosimeters (ionizing chambers) are used for screening purposes, whereas film dosimeters are used for regular surveillance.

Possible air pollution by radioactive substances is assessed by first passing the polluted air through appropriate sorbents (for gases and vapours) or filters (for particles) and then measuring the radioactivity of the sample collected.

Biological assessment

The methods for the biological assessment of exposure to radioactive substances are the same as those used for the biological assessment of exposure to their non-radioactive counterparts. They are used only when internal contamination with radioactive substances is suspected. The biological specimen (urine, blood, faeces, expired air, etc.) is selected in relation to the target organ of the toxic substance in question. Radioactivity is measured directly or after separation of the radioactive substance by radiochemical methods. There is also the possibility of measuring the content of some radionuclides directly by whole-body counters, scintillation detectors, etc.

Clinical effects

The harmful effects of irradiation may be somatic or genetic. Somatic effects develop directly in the irradiated individual, while the genetic effects appear in his or her progeny. The possible genetic effects resulting from occupational exposures are to a great extent still unknown.

Radiation effects may be either stochastic or non-stochastic. Stochastic effects are those whose probability of occurrence, though not necessarily their severity, is considered to be a function of the dose received; the dose in such cases is assumed to be without threshold. Thus, with increasing dose, the incidence of stochastic effects increase in the exposed population. It is accepted that genetic and carcinogenic effects are stochastic. The risk of increased incidence of malignant tumours induced by radiation is the main stochastic somatic risk.

The term non-stochastic is applied to somatic effects for which the severity of the effect varies with the dose and for which there is a threshold value. Examples include cataract, non-malignant skin damage, suppression of haematopoiesis, and damage to gametes leading to loss of fertility.

Acute effects

Whole-body irradiation. Irradiation of the whole body with over 1 Gy of penetrating radiation in a single exposure or over 1–2 days results in the so-called acute radiation syndrome, which is characterized by cell damage and death in the exposed tissues. Under current occupational conditions, such exposures are extremely rare, and are seen only in cases of accidents. Radiation doses of 0.05–0.25 Gy may not give rise to any symptoms, though there may be chromosomal damage detectable in peripheral lymphocytes. Exposure to higher doses of up to about 1 Gy does not lead to any symptoms, but in some individuals a small decrease in the number of white blood cells and platelets may be observed compared with pre-exposure values, especially if pre-exposure values were established on a group basis.

Doses of 1–2.5 Gy produce prodromal symptoms (nausea, vomiting, fatigue) and early haematological changes, particularly early lymphocytopenia and transient leukocytosis. After a latent phase, radiation-induced suppression of bone marrow leads to leukopenia, thrombopenia, and anaemia. Haemorrhage and infection are common. The ID_{50} in untreated subjects is about 3 Gy. Doses above 4 Gy cause severe acute radiation syndrome with gastrointestinal complications.

Local irradiation. Accidental exposure of parts of the body—usually of the hands in occupational exposure—is more frequent than whole-body irradiation. Immediately after irradiation, or within a few minutes of it, erythema develops, which is the primary skin reaction and which may be rather mild in the case of low-level exposure. Then, before the development of a second phase of symptoms, there is a latent period, the length of which is inversely related to the size of the dose—i.e., the higher the dose, the shorter the latent period. The second phase includes hyperaemia and oedema. From this stage onwards the course of the symptoms varies depending on the degree of exposure. If the exposure has been below 10 Gy, hyperaemia and oedema gradually diminish, but hyperpigmentation or depigmentation may develop. If the exposure has been greater than 20 Gy, the second phase develops after a shorter latent period, and is followed by the development of vesicles and ulcers. In cases of very high exposure (25–50 Gy), hyperaemia and oedema are followed by necrosis.

Chronic effects

Chronic radiation sickness may occur in individuals who have been repeatedly exposed to ionizing radiation over a long period (several years) during which the total cumulative dose has reached at least 1.5–4 Gy.

Mild forms are revealed by the presence of slight neuroregulatory disorders (slight imbalance of the autonomic nervous system, tendency towards arterial hypotension, tachycardia and sinus arrhythmia, dyskinesia of the intestine and the biliary tract, general excitability) and moderate and unstable leukopenia. In more advanced cases, the changes become more severe and stable. There is a further progression of autonomic nervous disorders, inhibition of the secretory function of the stomach, the appearance of clinical and electrocardiographic indications of dystrophic changes in the myocardium against a background of persistent arterial hypotension, signs of microstructural changes in the central nervous system, ovarian dysfunction (hypomenorrhoea and oligomenorrhoea) in women, bone marrow hypoplasia with persistent leukopenia (both granulocytopenia and lymphocytopenia), and less persistent thrombocytopenia. The development of anaemia is an unfavourable prognostic sign. In chronic radiation sickness caused by radioactive substances incorporated in the bone tissue, ostealgia may develop.

Chronic radiodermatitis may develop when the total radiation dose to the skin reaches at least 20–30 Gy. The manifestations are para-esthesia, disturbances of sensation, pain, itching, dryness of the skin, smooth lines on the palms and the surfaces of the terminal phalanges, and moderate dystrophy of the finger nails. After cumulative doses of the order of 40 Gy, painful cracks and focal hyperkeratosis and congestive hyperaemia appear. Late radiation ulcer may develop after cumulative doses of 50 Gy or more; this condition has a protracted course and the healing capacity of the body is distinctly reduced. Radiation carcinoma of the skin sometimes develops at injury sites.

Eye cataract may develop following exposure of the eye lens to large doses of X-rays, gamma-rays, and particularly, neutrons. This condition is characterized by the formation of a subcapsular radiation cataract at the posterior pole of the lens. While neutron radiation may induce lens opacities at a dose of only 0.5 Gy, doses of 6 Gy or more of X-rays are required at a single exposure to produce a similar effect. Eye cataract may also develop after long-term exposure, but the accumulated dose must be considerably higher. In its early stage, it can be easily distinguished from senile cataract. However, this is no longer possible if the nucleus of the lens is also affected.

Delayed effects

Carcinogenesis. A variety of cancers have been observed following exposure to ionizing radiation. The following types of cancer are related to occupational exposure:

Skin cancer (squamous cell) usually occurs after chronic radioder-matitis. Medical and dental practitioners who have worked in the past with radioactive substance, without adequate protection are most liable to such cancers.

Bone tumours are seen in radium dial painters and medical personnel responsibile for radium therapy. Radium accumulates in the bone matrix.

Leukaemias (myelogenous) occur mainly in radiologists.

Lung carcinomas are found in uranium and pitchblende miners. The causative agents are radon and its daughter products.

The period between exposure to ionizing radiation and the development of cancer may vary from a few years to several decades. It is not known whether a threshold dose exists below which cancers do not occur. Exposure limits for radiation exposure are based on the assumption that there is a linear, non-threshold relationship between dose level and the development of cancer. Epidemiological studies indicate that there is an increased incidence of the above type of cancers in occupational groups exposed to cumulative doses of several Gy. However, at lower doses and lower dose rates, the statistical probability of tumour development is so small that changes in cancer incidence under present working conditions (exposure levels) have not been found to be statistically significant in most cohort studies.

Exposure–effect relationship

The exposure–effect relationship has already been discussed under different preceding headings.

Prognosis

Acute effects of radiation caused by a dose up to 4 Gy have a favourable prognosis if they are treated properly.

The absence of early symptoms may indicate that the radiation dose did not exceed 1 Gy. Changes in the peripheral blood (extent and persistence of lymphocytopenia, high initial neutrophilic leukocytosis) during the first day are typical of heavier exposure (radiation dose exceeding 4 Gy). Early changes in arterial pressure and pulse rate, hyperthermia, and hyperbilirubinaemia occur in the extremely severe form of injury (radiation dose approximating to 10 Gy). Liquid stools for a short time during the first day are also an indication of severe irradiation of the intestines (radiation dose of the intestinal region exceeding 6–8 Gy). Finally, the appearance of erythema on the first day points to a high (> 4 Gy) local or whole-body irradiation.

Acute local injury resulting in ulcers and necrosis may lead to deformation and atrophy. In such cases it may become necessary to amputate the affected body part.

The prognosis of chronic radiation sickness is in general favourable and the manifestations improve or at least remain stable after the exposure has been terminated. Eye cataract and radiodermatitis are, however, irreversible. The prognosis of malignancies does not differ from that of tumours of other etiology.

Differential diagnosis

Some of the clinical manifestations of radiation effects (symptoms of acute exposure, early stages of cataract, acute and chronic radiodermatitis) have rather typical features. When there is clear evidence of radiation overexposure, the diagnosis can be made with certainty. The association between the other less specific or non-specific symptoms (particularly bone marrow suppression and cancers) and occupational exposure can be considered in individual cases only on the basis of probability. If there is evidence of heavy occupational exposure in the past, the probability that the cancer is related to occupational exposure is greatly increased.

Susceptibility

Post-radiation overexposure and diseases affecting organs sensitive to ionizing radiation may increase susceptibility. In some countries, work involving exposure to ionizing radiation is not permitted if the individual is suffering from any of the following conditions: haemoglobin less than 120 g/litre for women and 140 g/litre for men; persistent changes in the composition of the peripheral blood; haemorrhagic diathesis; mental disorders and diseases of the peripheral nervous system with pronounced functional inadequacy; drug addiction; obvious forms of neurosis; malignant tumours and precancerous diseases; organic diseases of the internal organs with frequent acute attacks; stage II hypertension; visual acuity below 0.6 for the better eye and below 0.5 for the other eye; and disseminated skin diseases.

There is no evidence of differences in susceptibility between men and women, but since the fetus may be more sensitive pregnant women need to be protected from ionizing radiation.

Health examinations

Preplacement examination

The preplacement examination should include a medical history and a physical examination, with special attention to the skin, eyes, and the respiratory system (in case of possible exposure to radioactive aerosols). A blood count should also be done.

Periodic examination

In medical terms, the periodic examination is the same as the preplacement one, and as a rule it should be carried out once a year. Additional examinations may also be necessary (e.g., after over-exposure or after radioactive contamination).

Workers whose exposure exceeds 30 % of the annual exposure limit require more detailed surveillance (including regular blood counts and tests of neurovascular function). Results of such examinations provide useful background information in treating accidental over-exposures and in detecting the presence of any conditions contraindicating further work involving ionizing radiation exposure. Exposures slightly higher than the exposure limits do not usually cause any detectable clinical injury and therefore clinical and medical observations are not considered appropriate for routine monitoring.

Case management

Acute radiation injuries require specialized treatment. After recovery, further exposure to ionizing radiation should be avoided. Persons who have recovered from chronic radiation sickness need not necessarily be transferred from their jobs if the working conditions have been improved in the meantime and if the radiation levels are well below the exposure limits.

If in any worker the established annual exposure limit is exceeded and there are no detectable adverse effects, the worker should still be removed temporarily from radiation exposure in order to permit his average cumulative dose to fall below the established limit.

In the case of external contamination with radionuclides, the contaminant must be removed as soon as possible in order to prevent internal contamination. Internal contamination requires specialized treatment to speed up the elimination of the radionuclide from the body.

Control measures

Exposure to radiation from both sealed sources (e.g., X-ray equipment, nuclear power plants) and unsealed sources (e.g., radioactive chemicals in medical and industrial laboratories) can be controlled by: (*a*) reducing the duration of exposure; (*b*) maintaining a safe distance between the worker and the source of radiation (the intensity of radiation varies inversely with the square of the distance from the radiation source); and (*c*) shielding the radiation source with materials that absorb ionizing radiation (e.g., lead). It is recommended that all radiation sources should be kept covered with shields, and personal protection devices (such as lead-rubber gloves and aprons) should always be used during work involving radiation exposure.

In the case of unsealed sources of ionizing radiation, there is an additional danger of internal contamination; good personal hygiene should therefore, be strictly enforced. The control measures for different radioactive substances vary from the simple application of general rules of safe laboratory work to completely enclosing work processes, depending on the physical state of the substance (solid, liquid, gaseous), the amount, and chemical and radioactive toxicity.

Exposure limits for ionizing radiation have been recommended jointly by ILO, WHO, IAEA, and NEA.[1] For the control of stochastic effects, the annual *effective dose-equivalent*[2] *limit* is 50 mSv (5 rem). For non-stochastic effects, the annual *dose-equivalent limit* for individual organs and tissues is 500 mSv (50 rem), except for the eye lens, for which the limit is 150 mSv (15 rem). In terms of radiation dose, the internal exposure limits are the same as those for external exposure. The limits on intake may be calculated for individual radioactive substances on the basis of their radioactivity.

Pregnant women should not be subjected to annual exposures exceeding 30% of the dose-equivalent limits.

---

[1] Basic safety standards for radiation protection. Vienna, International Atomic Energy Agency, 1982 (Report of an advisory group jointly sponsored by IAEA/WHO/ILO/NEA).

[2] The *dose-equivalent* is the product of the absorbed dose (in Gy) and the quality factor of the type of ionizing radiation (e.g., 1 for X-rays, 10 for neutrons, and 20 for alpha-particles). The unit of dose-equivalent is the sievert (Sv), and 1 Sv = 1 J kg = 100 rem. The *effective dose-equivalent* corresponds to the mean dose-equivalent in a tissue modified by a weighting factor reflecting the detriment from stochastic effects.

CHAPTER 27

Occupational skin diseases[1]

Properties of the causal agents

The number of possible causal agents is very large, and only major classes of common hazards can be mentioned here.

Physical agents. These include pressure or friction, weather conditions (wind, rain, frost, sun), heat, radiation (ultraviolet, ionizing), and mineral fibres.

Chemical agents. These are further divided into four categories:

(*a*) primary irritants—acids, alkalis, lipid solvents, detergents, metallic salts (of arsenic, mercury, etc.), etc;

(*b*) sensitizers[2]—metals and their salts (chromium, nickel, cobalt, etc.), compounds derived from aniline (*p*-phenylenediamine, azodyes, etc.), aromatic nitroderivatives (trinitrotoluene, etc.), resins (particularly monomers and additives such as epoxyresins, formaldehyde, vinyls, acrylics, accelerators, plasticizers), rubber chemicals (vulcanizers such as dimethyl thiuram disulfide, antioxidants, etc.), drugs and antibiotics (e.g., procaine, phenothiazines, chlorothiazide, penicillin, and tetracycline), cosmetics, turpentine, plants (e.g., primula and chrysanthemum), etc;

(*c*) acnegenic agents—chlorinated naphthalenes and bifenyls, mineral oils, etc; and

(*d*) photosensitizers—anthracene, pitch, aminobenzoic acid derivatives, chlorinated aromatic hydrocarbons, acridine dyes, etc.

Biological agents. Several microorganisms (microbes, fungi), skin parasites, and their products also cause skin diseases.

Occurrence and uses

Most of the possible agents occur in industrial work. Exposure to weather conditions is common among those who work in the open air e.g., agricultural workers and sailors). Some of the chemical agents may occur as undesirable contaminants of other chemicals or industrial

---

[1] This chapter includes skin diseases caused by physical, chemical or biological agents not included under other items.

[2] Almost all chemicals can act as sensitzers. The chemicals included here are some of the more potent ones.

byproducts (e.g., chromium in cement production and tetrachloro-benzodioxine in pentachlorophenol synthesis).

Occupations involving exposure to agents causing skin diseases

Some of the most exposed groups are: agricultural workers (weather conditions, plants, zoonotic agents, pesticides, antibiotics or other animal food additives, etc.); construction material production workers (cement, etc.); construction workers (cement, mineral fibres, paints, plastics, etc.); chemical production workers (types of exposure according to the substances present); electroplaters (degreasers, acids, metallic salts); dyers; glass-reinforced plastics production workers (mineral fibres, resins); painters (dyes, metallic salts, solvents, etc.); workers in engineering industries (cutting oils or lubricants, etc.); health personnel (drugs, antibiotics, local anaesthetics, disinfectants, etc.); animal dealers; and butchers (zoonotic agents).

Mechanisms of action

Physical agents cause direct mechanical, thermal or radiation injury to the skin. Similarly, most of the irritants damage skin directly by: (a) altering its pH; (b) reacting with its proteins (denaturation); (c) extracting lipids from its outer layer; or (d) lowering skin resistance. Reaction-producing skin allergy is mostly a delayed type of hypersensitivity reaction. The sensitizing agent combines with protein in the epidermis to form a hapten-protein complex, against which antibodies are produced. Acnegenic agents block the sebaceous glands and ducts, causing local inflammation. Photosensitizers increase the sensitivity of skin to ultraviolet radiation.

Assessment of exposure

Occupational skin diseases result from direct contact of the skin with the causal agent. Thus, work history and clear evidence of the presence of the agent in question in the material handled by the worker is essential for the assessment of exposure.

Clinical effects

Primary irritant contact dermatitis is the most frequently encountered occupational dermatosis. The acute form is characterized by erythema, oedema, papules, vesicles or bullae, localized as a rule on the hands, forearms or face. A skin patch test with the causal agent can induce and confirm irritative effects and the etiology of the dermatosis. The manifestations of chronic irritant contact dermatitis are similar to those of many other dermatoses, such as chronic allergic contact eczema, hyperkeratosis, etc. Whereas the causal agent of acute irritant dermatitis is usually obvious, in chronic dermatitis the etiological factor is mostly inconspicuous. The lesions are often caused by detergents, weak alkalis, organic solvents, or less potent or diluted chemicals so that their effect is delayed, i.e., it appears only after the resistance capacity of the skin has been exhausted.

In addition to their direct effects, primary irritants can render the skin vulnerable to infection and injury, particularly injury by sensitizing agents.

Allergic contact dermatitis (eczema) (both acute and chronic) has the same clinical features as non-occupational eczema. The acute form resembles acute irritant dermatitis and the chronic form is character- ized by lichenification and fissuring. Patch tests are helpful in diagnosing skin hypersensitivity. (The patch test involves the application of a non-irritating concentration of the suspected allergen to a part of the unaffected skin of the patient for 24–48 hours; in positive cases, an eczematous dermatitis develops beneath the covering patch.)

Occupational acne is characterized by plugged sebaceous follicles and suppurative lesions. While the acne caused by mineral oil or tar and pitch affect only those sites of the body that come into close contact with the agent, that caused by chlorinated aromatic compounds may be more generalized.

Microtraumatic lesions are caused by natural or man-made mineral fibres (glass or other silicates), and are characterized by tiny whitish or pink papules localized on the exposed sites, particularly on the arms.

Acute solar dermatosis is regarded as an occupational disease if it is largely promoted by photodynamic substances used in the occupation—e.g., tar and tar-derived products, sulfonamides, pheno- thiazines, or tetracyclines.

Skin diseases caused by ionizing radiation are discussed in Chapter 26.

Skin cancers of occupational origin (squamous or basal cell carcinoma, rarely other types) do not differ from other similar non- occupational tumours (see Chapter 28). Histological examinations are useful in defining the exact type of the tumour, but they do indicate the etiology. Occupational tumours tend to occur on the skin surface most exposed to the carcinogens and develop from precancerous lesions (hyperkeratosis, papillomatosis).

The most frequent *contagious occupational skin diseases* are zoonotic diseases: dermatophytoses, candidiasis, erysipeloid, tuberculosis ver- rucosa, etc. (see also Chapter 29).

Exposure–effect relationship

The extent and severity of contact irritant dermatitis, acne and radiation-induced diseases vary with the degree of exposure. On the other hand, allergic contact dermatitis (eczema) can be induced even by minute amounts of allergens.

Prognosis

Irritant dermatitis, acne, and infectious diseases heal after the causative agent has been removed. (For details of radiation-induced dermatitis see Chapter 26). The prognosis of allergic eczema depends on the nature of the allergen and the duration of the affection. If the patient is removed from the exposure early and if exposure to the allergen is confined to the workplace, full recovery is the rule. However, if the allergen is also widespread in the general environment (e.g., chromium, detergents, etc.), or if secondary allergy to bacterial infection in the eczematous lesions develops, the skin affection may last throughout life.

Differential diagnosis

The clinical picture of most occupational skin diseases is similar to that of their non-occupational counterparts. The differential diagnosis is based on two principles: (a) proper diagnosis of the nosological entity in order to exclude immediately diseases of non-occupational origin (e.g., palmar psoriasis, hyperkeratosis, mycosis, or contact allergic eczema); (b) identification of the etiological agent of occupational dermatoses (e.g., differentiating contact allergic eczema due to occupational exposure to epoxy resins from eczema due to hypersensitivity to turpentine in shoe-polish used at home).

The following general guidelines should be followed in the diagnosis of occupational skin diseases:

—The clinical picture, localization, and the course of the disease must correspond fully to the established characteristics of the occupational disease.
—Occupational exposure to the harmful agent must be proved with certainty.
—There must be a reasonable time relationship between the development of the skin disease and the onset of exposure to the suspected agent (i.e., a latent period—incubation time in infectious diseases, development of sensitization in eczema).
—In contact allergic dermatitis (eczema), patch tests should give positive results and confirmation may be obtained by other types of laboratory examination.

—There should be a positive response to removal from work and re-exposure. As a rule the affection improves during absence from work (e.g., during holidays, and relapses after return to work). It should also be noted that non-occupational eczema may deteriorate at the workplace owing to possible nonspecific irritation.

—The development of a skin disease in a group of workers usually indicates that the disease is of occupational etiology.

—Any non-occupational cause of the disease must be excluded, e.g., chemicals or other allergens or irritants at home, substances encountered in leisure activities and drugs.

Susceptibility

Persons with atopy (eczema and other allergic skin diseases and also allergic affections of other organs), chronic skin affections including hyperhidrosis, seborrhoea or ichthyosis, abnormal pigmentation, and precancerous skin lesions are more susceptible than others.

Health examinations

Preplacement examination

The preplacement examination should include a medical history and a physical examination, with special attention to the skin (of the whole body) and allergies (atopy).

Periodic examination

In medical terms the periodic examination is the same as the preplacement one. Patch tests are not recommended for the screening of symptom-free subjects. Intervals between examinations usually range from 6 months to 2 years, depending on the level of exposure at the workplace.

Case management

Patients with occupational allergic contact dermatitis (eczema) almost always require transfer to another workplace free of the causal allergens. Patients with irritative dermatitis and other acute non-allergic affections should be temporarily removed from exposure, and should be allowed to return to their original jobs only after the causal agent has been controlled. Permanent transfer to another job may be necessary in the case of subjects in whom repeated temporary transfers do not lead to a complete recovery. Precancerous conditions require permanent removal from exposure to the causal agent.

Control measures

Whenever possible, strong allergens, sensitizers, and carcinogens should be replaced by less dangerous substances. Skin contact with causal agents should be limited by technical control measures; the key to effective prevention is the elimination of skin contact with them. Protective clothing, aprons, gloves or barrier creams, boots, and face masks may be necessary. Basic facilities for personal cleanliness (showers, etc.) should be provided, and their use should be encouraged or made mandatory.

CHAPTER 28

Primary epitheliomatous cancer of the skin

This chapter deals with primary epitheliomatous cancer of the skin caused by tar, pitch, mineral oil, anthracene, and compounds, products, and residues of these substances.

Properties of the causal agents

Tar (or coal-tar) is a distillation product of coal. Pitches are of different types, and may be produced by the distillation of either coal or crude petroleum. The term mineral oil refers to petroleum and other hydrocarbon oils obtained from mineral sources. Anthracene is a distillation product of coal-tar. All these substances and their cancer-producing derivatives are complex mixtures in which the actual carcinogens are probably polycyclic aromatic hydrocarbons. They also contain a number of tumour-promoting compounds.

Tar is a brownish, viscous substance, and pitch is a heavy, viscid, dark-brown material. The derivatives of these substances may be liquid, solid, or vapour. As a general rule, bitumens derived from petroleum are much less carcinogenic than tars derived from coal.

Occurrence and uses

Carcinogenic products of carbonaceous materials are present in coal-tars and pitch, heavy tar oils, certain mineral oils, products of coking operations, soot, creosote oil, crude paraffins, and shale oil and its distillation and fractionation products. These substances have many uses as indicated in the section below.

Occupations involving the risk of epitheliomatous cancer

The following workers are at risk of developing primary epitheliomatous cancer of the skin: tar distillers; coal-gas manufacturers; coke plant workers; fishing net and rope makers; briquette manufacturers; caulking material manufacturers; roofers, road builders (exposure to pitch and tar products); shale oil workers and refinery workers; match factory, naphthalene, paper industry, and munitions

194

workers exposed to crude paraffins; ship stokers; carbon black makers; chimney sweeps (exposure to soot); and timber picklers (exposure to creosote oil).

Mechanism of action

Long-term repeated exposure to tars and related substances appears to cause cancer, predominantly at the site of contact with the skin. Metabolic activation of polycyclic aromatic hydrocarbons appears to play some role in their carcinogenicity.

Cancer may also develop as a result of a possible synergistic effect of polycyclic hydrocarbon carcinogens and ultraviolet radiation.

Assessment of exposure

Environmental assessment

The concentrations of polycyclic aromatic hydrocarbons in coal-tars and related materials and in air samples may be used to assess the toxicity of different substances and the level of exposure to polycyclic aromatic hydrocarbons at the workplace.

Routine methods to quantify contact of such substances with the skin are not currently available.

Fluorescent substances in tars on the skin may be detected under ultra violet light. If performed, this procedure must be undertaken judiciously in order to avoid a photosensitivity reaction.

Biological assessment

Useful procedures are not currently available.

Clinical effects

Erythema accompanied by a burning sensation ("pitch smarts") usually appears within a few hours or days of exposure at the site of contact with coal-tar, pitch, etc. The burning sensation is intensified by exposure of the affected parts to sunlight. After repeated exposure over several years, thickening of the skin, hyperpigmentation, comedones (blackheads), and follicular inflammation may occur. Conjunctivitis is common, and is often accompanied by photophobia.

Long-term exposure causes chronic skin changes, which include:

—irregular areas of atrophy;
—patchy hyperpigmentation and hypopigmentation;
—wart-like papillomas (particularly on damaged skin), some of which may later develop into squamous cell cancers; and
—basal cell carcinomas and keratocanthomas.

The scrotum is particularly prone to develop squamous cell cancers following exposure to tar and soot. Skin cancers usually take 5–50 years or more to develop, and may occur even after the cessation of exposure.

Inhalation of dusts and vapours of tar, pitches, etc. has been reported to cause tumours of the lung.

Exposure–effect relationship

Owing to a paucity of data, the exposure–effect relationship is not yet established.

Prognosis

The prognosis is good if lesions are detected and treated before extensive invasion occurs.

Differential diagnosis

The pathological identity of suspected epitheliomatous cancers can be confirmed by biopsy and histological examinations. Occupational and non-occupational causes must be differentiated.

Susceptibility

Factors contributing to increased susceptibility have not yet been established with certainty.

Health examinations

Preplacement examination

A medical history and a physical examination are necessary to ensure that precancerous conditions (e.g., keratoses) or skin cancers are not present.

Periodic examination

Regular examination of skin ensures early detection and treatment of premalignant and malignant lesions. It is sufficient to carry out such examinations at one-year intervals.

Case management

Premalignant and malignant skin lesions should be treated promptly in order to avoid progression. In individuals who develop lesions, removal from further exposure must be considered, especially in the case of cancers associated with polycyclic aromatic hydrocarbons. Failing this, very careful attention must be given to control measures.

Control measures

Whenever possible, tars and related substances should be replaced by non-carcinogenic materials. Technical control measures should be applied to reduce air and surface contamination. Work clothes should be kept separate from other clothes and should be washed and changed regularly. Impervious protective clothing such as gloves, smocks, and worksuits should be used whenever necessary. Finally, workers should be made aware of the hazards associated with work involving exposure to tars, pitches, etc. and of the protective measures recommended above.

As far as possible, workers exposed to polycyclic aromatic hydrocarbons should avoid exposure to ultravoilet light during and soon after work.

CHAPTER 29

Infectious and parasitic diseases

Properties of the causal agents

Exposure to live infective microorganisms and parasites and their toxic products is encountered in many occupations. The most important agents of occupation-related infectious and parasitic diseases are: (*a*) viruses (viral hepatitis, Newcastle virus disease, rabies); (*b*) chlamydiae and rickettsiae (ornithosis, Q fever, tickborne rickettsiosis); (*c*) bacteria (anthrax, brucellosis (undulant fever), erysipeloid, leptospirosis (Weil's disease), tetanus, tuberculosis, tularaemia, wound sepsis); (*d*) fungi (candidiasis and dermatophytosis of the skin and mucous membranes, coccidiomycosis, histoplasmosis); (*e*) protozoa (leishmaniasis, malaria, trypanosomiasis); and (*f*) helminths (hookworm disease, schistosomiasis).

The survival and pathogenicity of these agents in the working environment are largely determined by: physical and climatic factors (temperature, humidity, oxygen tension, soil conditions), nutritional and other requirements for multiplication, and, in the case of parasites, presence of obligatory reservoirs and vectors, which are mostly animals.

Occurrence

Work-related infectious and parasitic diseases are mostly encountered in:

—agricultural work;
—certain workplaces in warmer and less developed countries;
—hospitals, laboratories, clinics, autopsy rooms, etc.;
—work involving handling of animals and their products (veterinary clinics, slaughterhouses, meat and fish markets, etc.);
—outdoor work where animal excreta may be encountered (work in canals, rivers, ditches, sewers, docks, farm yards, construction sites, etc.).

Occupations involving exposure to infectious and parasitic diseases

Table 3 summarizes infectious and parasitic diseases encountered in different occupations.

Table 3. Summary of occupations and associated infectious and parasitic
diseases

Occupation	Diseases
Agriculture, animal husbandry, forestry, trapping, and hunting	In both tropical and temperate areas: anthrax, arthropod-borne viral diseases (e.g., encephalitis, plague), coccidiomycosis, fungal infections, histoplasmosis, leptospirosis, Q fever, rabies, tickborne rickettsiosis, tuberculosis, and tularaemia In tropical areas only: arthropod-borne viral diseases (e.g., yellow fever, haemorrhagic fever), hookworm, leishmaniasis, malaria, schistosomiasis, trypanosomiasis
Construction work, land excavation, sewer work, ditching, mining	Coccidiomycosis, hookworm, histoplasmosis, leptospirosis, tetanus, wound sepsis
Meat and fish handling and packing	Bovine tuberculosis, brucellosis, erysipeloid, fungal infections, Q fever, tularaemia
Poultry and bird handling	Fungal infections, Newcastle virus disease, ornithosis
Work with hair, hides, wool	Anthrax, Q fever
Veterinarians	Tuberculosis, brucellosis, fungal infections, leptospirosis, Newcastle virus disease, ornithosis, Q fever, rabies, tularaemia
Physicians, nurses, dentists, laboratory technicians	Viral hepatitis, tuberculosis, other communicable infections
Work in warm, humid conditions, (kitchens, gymnasiums, swimming pools, etc.)	Fungal infections of the skin

Mechanism of action

Infection occurs when an unimmunized or non-resistant person comes into contact with an infective agent. The mode of entry and pathophysiology of different diseases vary considerably. While some agents are able to penetrate intact skin (anthrax, brucellosis, leptospirosis, schistosomiasis, tularaemia), others require the skin to be damaged (erysipeloid, rabies, sepsis, tetanus, viral hepatitis B) or macerated (fungal infections). Some protozoan pathogens enter the body through insect bites (leishmaniasis, malaria, tickborne rickettsiosis, trypanosomiasis). Infection may also occur by the inhalation of droplets, spores, or contaminated dust (coccidiomycosis, histoplasmosis, Newcastle virus disease, ornithosis, Q fever, tuberculosis). Agents of viral hepatitis A, diarrhoeal diseases, and enteroviral diseases such as poliomyelitis enter the body through ingestion of contaminated food and water.

Some diseases result from an inflammatory reaction to toxins (endotoxins and exotoxins) produced by bacteria during reproduction.

Assessment of exposure

Assessment of the risk of exposure to infectious and parasitic diseases is only rarely feasible—e.g., search for encephalitis virus in ticks or for rabies virus in wild animals. However, the risk of a potential hazard in a group of workers can be assessed from:

—reports of cases of communicable or zoonotic diseases in groups of workers regarded as being at risk of contracting those diseases;

—epidemiological data on the incidence of communicable or zoonotic diseases;

—data on the prevalence of vectors and parasites;

—serological data on immunity status of workers (e.g., from serological or skin tests for tuberculosis and viral, rickettsial, chlamydial, and salmonella infections).

Clinical effects and diagnosis

Early signs of infections are seldom specific, but are usually sufficiently definite to warrant suspicion of disease if appropriate geographical and occupational factors are also present. Table 4 summarizes the early symptoms of infectious and parasitic diseases and possible corresponding diagnoses.

For full descriptions, diagnostic methods, differential diagnoses, prognoses, and treatment procedures of these diseases the reader is referred to standard medical textbooks.

Susceptibility

Individuals considered as being susceptible to infectious and parasitic diseases include: unimmunized persons; those recovering from serious systemic infections; those suffering from immunosuppression; and persons whose nutritional and general health status is poor.

Persons with renal and liver dysfunction are at increased risk of contracting leptospirosis and serum hepatitis. Minor injuries may increase the risk of skin infections, tetanus, rabies, and serum hepatitis. Wet or sweaty skin is more liable to attack by fungal infections; and anaerobic conditions resulting from puncture wounds and tissue destruction favour the multiplication of *Clostridium tetani*.

Table 4.   Early symptoms of infectious diseases and possible corresponding diagnoses

Early symptoms	Possible diagnoses
Severe illness with bad headache and symptoms of nervous system involvement	Brucellosis, leptospirosis, malaria, rabies, tickborne rickettsiosis, or trypanosomiasis
Fever with respiratory problems or pneumonia	Coccidiomycosis, histoplasmosis, ornithosis, Q fever, or tuberculosis
Severe systemic symptoms preceded by a skin lesion or ulcer	Anthrax, leishmaniasis, trypanosomiasis, or tularaemia
Gastrointestinal symptoms followed by dark urine and jaundice	Viral or leptospiral hepatitis
Painful muscular spasms, particularly around the jaw[a]	Tetanus
Progressive debility and anaemia, especially if preceded or accompanied by haematuria or blood-stained diarrhoea	Schistosomiasis
Indolent itching and erythematous skin lesions	Erysipeloid (if on hands), hookworm (if on feet), or fungal or bacterial infection (if skin appears to be damaged or macerated)

[a] Note that if tetanus is not suspected at this stage it is easily missed.

Health examinations

The vast majority of persons exposed to infectious and parasitic diseases are self-employed rural workers in developing countries. Since they mostly live and work in areas that are not readily accessible, health examinations are rarely, if ever, done. However, certain groups of workers in rural areas (health workers, municipal workers, construction and mining workers, etc.) can be reached more easily and regular health examinations of such workers should be encouraged.

Moreover, in certain areas it may be possible to identify groups of rural workers at risk of contracting a particular disease; in such cases regular health examinations will be particularly useful. Whenever possible, health examinations should be promoted among rural workers.

Preplacement examination

The preplacement examination should include a medical history and a physical examination. The main objectives of this examination are: (a) to determine and record initial health status of the worker; (b) to identify susceptible persons; and (c) to diagnose and treat latent and active cases of infectious diseases. In occupations involving the risk of tuberculosis (e.g., health service workers and veterinary and laboratory workers), the tuberculin test should also be done along with a chest X-ray. Depending on the geographical area and occupation, selected serological and microbiological tests may also be necessary in order to detect past or current infection. Whenever possible, all workers should be immunized against locally prevalent diseases for which vaccinations exist.

Periodic examination

In medical terms, the periodic examination is the same as the preplacement one. It involves the maintenance of medical records of febrile or infective illnesses by systematic inquiry and by repetition of previously conducted serological tests; in tuberculin-positive workers, a chest X-ray should be repeated.

In most rural workers, periodic examinations are desirable at annual intervals; in the case of health and laboratory workers, the interval should be 6 months.

Case management

Cases of infectious and parasitic diseases should be notified at once to the appropriate health authority. Specific antibiotic treatment or chemotherapy is fairly effective in most but not all diseases. The success of the treatment will depend on correct diagnosis and skilled care. Cases of tetanus should be treated urgently in well-equipped hospitals. Isolation of patients with contagious diseases may be necessary.

Control measures

Environmental

Some zoonoses can be controlled by eliminating their animal reservoirs or insect vectors. Spraying of residual insecticides may be used against mosquitos (larvae as well as adults), sandflies, and tsetse flies. Predatory fish can reduce the population of snails, that harbour schistosoma parasites, and rodent control is useful against leptospirosis. The immunization of cattle and domestic animals is an effective way of reducing the risk of brucellosis and rabies, respectively. By controlling and restricting the import of birds, domestic mammals, hides, wool, and products made from animal bone it may be possible to prevent ornithosis, psittacosis (parrot fever), and anthrax. In certain workplaces, dust suppression by exhaust ventilation may also prevent airborne anthrax and ornithosis.

Protection of workers

Health education

Exposed groups should be informed about the nature of infectious and parasitic hazards in their occupation and region. Special emphasis should be placed on personal hygiene and workers should be urged to wear appropriate protective clothing (especially boots and shoes), handle animals and animal products with care, avoid swimming and wading in contaminated water, avoid drinking unboiled milk, and protect themselves from animal and insect bites.

Specific prophylaxis

All workers should be vaccinated against tetanus, especially those working in agriculture. Other vaccines should be used as required: BCG for tuberculin-negative health workers; rabies and anthrax vaccines for veterinarians; typhus and Q fever vaccines for laboratory workers and populations in endemic areas. Chemoprophylaxis with suppressive drugs is important for workers in malarious areas. Immunoglobulins may be useful in providing passive protection in cases of injuries and in unimmunized persons at risk of developing tetanus, rabies, or hepatitis B.

Protective clothing

Gloves and boots should be worn by all persons working in mines, rivers, ditches, fields, etc. where there is risk of schistosomiasis, leptospirosis, and hookworm. Gloves and barrier creams are also useful in protecting animal and fish handlers from fungal infections and erysipeloid. Laboratory and certain health service employees may also require special protective clothing.

Codes of practice

Ideally, such codes are required for all occupations exposed to infectious agents, but at present they exist only for workers in laboratories and autopsy rooms, some groups of sewer workers, abattoir and animal product workers, and hospital staff (for protection against viral hepatitis). Codes for hospital staff include screening of blood donors, blood recipients and hospital staff for hepatitis B antigen, rules for the sterilization and disposal of instruments and contaminated materials, and the provision of separate facilities for dialysis and other surgical procedures for virus carriers.

Clinical and laboratory tests for the early detection of occupational diseases in the main organs and systems

CHAPTER 30

The respiratory system

Function

The exchange of carbon dioxide and oxygen between blood and air takes place in the alveolar parts of the lungs. The exchange is regulated by the rate and depth of reciprocal airflow (breathing) and depends on the diffusion of oxygen from alveoli into the blood in capillaries in the alveolar walls. The same is true also for inhaled gases and vapours. The lungs represent the most important route of entry of airborne hazardous substances in occupational exposure.

Pathophysiological mechanisms

Strongly irritant gases, aerosols, and dusts cause reflex coughing or laryngeal spasm (cessation of breathing). If these substances penetrate deep into the lungs, toxic bronchitis, lung oedema or pneumonitis may develop. Workers become tolerant to low levels of irritant exposure by increasing mucus secretion, a mechanism characteristic of bronchitis and also seen in tobacco smokers.

Dust and aerosol particles greater than 15 μm in diameter are filtered out in the upper airways. Particles of 5–15 μm are caught on the lower airway lining and moved back up to the larynx by mucociliary action. They may then be swallowed. Particles in this size range that irritate the airways or release substances provoking an immune response may cause respiratory diseases, such as bronchitis.

Particles between 0.5 and 5 μm in diameter (respirable dust) may pass beyond the mucociliary clearance system and enter the terminal airways and alveoli. From there they are collected by scavenger cells (macrophages) and transported back to the mucociliary system or into the lymphatic system. Particles less than 0.5 μm in diameter probably remain suspended in the air and are not retained. Elongated particles or fibres less than 3 μm in diameter and up to 100 μm in length may reach the terminal airways, but are not removed by the macrophages; they may, however, be engulfed by more than one macrophage and become coated with an iron-rich protein material resulting in the characteristic "asbestos" bodies.

The main causes of respiratory diseases are:

(a) pathogenic microorganisms that survive phagocytosis;

(b) mineral particles that cause damage or death of the macrophage that engulfs them, both preventing clearance and provoking a tissue reaction;

(c) organic particles that provoke an immune response;

(d) overload of the system by sustained exposure to high concentrations of respirable dust that accumulate around the terminal airways.

Repeated stimulation of the airways (perhaps even by inert particles), leads to thickening of the walls of the bronchi, increased secretion of mucus, lowering of threshold to reflex narrowing and coughing, increased susceptibility to respiratory infection, and asthmatic symptoms.

Organic dusts (and some chemical substances such as isocyanates and platinum) may provoke an immune response with reversible narrowing of the airways (immediate or delayed), sometimes causing persistent narrowing in susceptible individuals.

The lung periphery is damaged particularly by fibrogenic dust. Most fibrogenic particles entering the lungs are partially cleared and deposited on the hilar lymph nodes. There, the particles provoke a tissue reaction, thickening and scarring the nodes in the process. This obstructs lymphatic drainage and causes the particles entering the lungs as a result of further exposure to accumulate near the scarred nodes, progressively enlarging the scarred area. Vascular thrombosis in the perivascular lymphatics and lung necrosis result in progressive fibrosis in the septa, leading to stiffening of the lung. Scarring in these various ways leads to contraction of the damaged lung and overstretching of the remaining lung, uneven ventilation, and certain types of emphysema.

Common disorders and differential diagnosis

The disorders depend mainly on the type of agent: inert dust, fibrogenic dust; chemical irritants, allergens, and carcinogens.

Inert dust

Even relatively inert dusts exert some effects. The main effects of inert dust are:

(a) *Increased load on bronchopulmonary clearance.* This causes increased secretion of mucus, bronchial transport of the mucus with expectoration, and finally cough with phlegm.

(b) *Obstructive changes in lung function.* These include slight decrease in forced expiratory volume in one second ($FEV_{1.0}$), slight decrease in vital capacity (VC), and increase in intrathoracic gas volume. The changes are detectable epidemiologically (changes in group values); most individual values remain in the normal range.

The role of inert dust exposure in the development of airflow limitation (obstructive respiratory disease) at concentrations currently present in the workplaces in industrialized countries remains to be clarified. The effect of inert dust is difficult to distinguish, in individual cases, from infective and obstructive bronchitis of other types (e.g., due to smoking).

Tests for the detection of airflow limitation (including those for the diseases of the small airways) should be included in periodic health examinations of workers exposed to high dust concentrations. The tests include: forced expiratory volume in one second ($FEV_{1.0}$), ventilatory capacity (VC), flow resistance test (for large airway function), maximum mid-expiratory flow (MMF), maximum expiratory flow at 25 % or 50 % of ventilatory capacity ($V_{max_{25}}$, $V_{max_{50}}$), and closing volume test (for small airway function).

Fibrogenic dust

Quartz-containing dust causes silicosis. The X-ray changes must be distinguished from other diseases causing dispersed shadows (e.g., tuberculosis and sarcoidosis). Even large opacities on the X-ray may be accompanied by fairly small loss of lung function in those suffering from silicosis of the restrictive type. In advanced cases of anthracosis with large opacities (type A, B or C according to the ILO *International Classification of Radiographs of Pneumoconioses*), airways obstruction is normally found.

As in workers exposed to inert dust, lung function tests suitable for the early detection of airway obstruction should be used. The importance of this examination is underlined by the fact that obstructive respiratory diseases of non-occupational origin (allergic, viral, bacterial, etc.) are very frequent and can invariably be successfully controlled if detected early enough.

Asbestos-containing dust typically causes restrictive lung function impairment (i.e., decrease of VC and intrathoracic gas volume and lung compliance) but with high normal relative $FEV_{1.0}$ value ($FEV_{1.0}/VC \times 100$) and flow resistance values. Diffusing capacity is invariably impaired early in the course of disease, as is inspiratory capacity. The early detection of impairment preceding X-ray changes in individuals is possible only by regular periodic examinations, otherwise only group-based changes are detectable.

Chemical irritants

Long-term exposure to various irritant chemical substances may cause symptoms of bronchitis, such as cough with or without sputum or wheezing. The symptoms may or may not be accompanied by increased bronchial reactivity. High-level exposures (as a rule in accidents) can cause severe acute bronchitis (often haemorrhagic) with airway obstruction and/or pulmonary oedema. Lung function impairment of the restrictive type may develop as a result of acute damage if alveolar oedema is present (e.g., from exposure to zinc fumes). This impairment is usually transitory and settles in several months. Other exposures (e.g., to oxides of nitrogen), may result in permanent damage of the small airways.

In health supervision of workers exposed to chemical irritants, tests for the detection of airflow limitation (in large and/or small airways) and of bronchial reactivity may prove useful. However, in most cases, medical history and physical examination give earlier indications of incipient health impairment than do lung function tests because there may be no detectable functional impairment in cases of non-obstructive bronchitis.

Allergens

These include organic materials of animal or vegetable origin, (e.g., fungal spores) and probably certain chemicals (e.g., platinum salts). Early detection of allergic respiratory reactions is of major importance because by eliminating further exposure to allergens and by appropriate early treatment full recovery, or at least a symptom-free course of the disease, is possible. It may not be easy to distinguish between idiopathic asthma and other immunological disorders. The significance of the signs of general sensitization prior to the development of manifest disease of the respiratory system should be considered. For differential diagnosis, tests of general sensitization (e.g., skin scarification and/or intracutaneous tests, histamine liberation in blood), organ-bound sensitization (conjunctival test, intranasal test or inhalation test), and inhalatory tests for bronchial reactivity may give important information.

Hypersensitivity reactions to allergens may be tested by simulating workplace exposures in the laboratory or by inhalatory provocative tests. The air concentration of the allergen in such tests should correspond to that occurring in the workplace.

Sometimes allergic or immunological reactions may manifest themselves as attacks of alveolitis with fever and lung infiltration. However, these acute attacks may not be detected clinically, and after further exposure to allergens, they may develop into lung fibrosis with restrictive type of lung function impairment. The detection of lung function changes does not necessarily mean that changes will be found on the X-rays. The determination of VC, lung compliance, and intrathoracic gas volume and diffusing capacity can facilitate the diagnosis of the early stages of respiratory damage.

Carcinogens

Asbestos and uranium dusts are the best known examples of agents causing occupational lung cancer. The role of tobacco smoking both as a causative and as a synergistic factor (in exposure to asbestos) has been well established.

Carcinogenic properties of agents found in workplaces can be detected by epidemiological studies. Unfortunately, there are no efficient methods for the early detection of lung cancer.

Clinical examinations and tests

Chest radiography

Standard-distance, full-size, postero-anterior films taken and processed as recommended by ILO[1] play an important role in the prevention and early detection of occupational diseases of the alveolar part of the lung.

For epidemiological purposes, the classification of individual X-rays of pneumoconiosis is a difficult task and even those experienced in radiography vary considerably in their judgement. In general, rounded opacities are fairly specific for pneumoconiosis due to mineral dusts. Other changes such as irregular opacities (which are frequently seen after exposure to asbestos dust) are less specific.

In exposure–response epidemiological studies, it is recommended that random groups of X-rays be examined by at least three experienced medical workers independently, using standard ILO X-rays for comparison. In order to ensure repeatability, a certain number of X-rays should be re-examined, and use should be made of trigger films. However, it should be pointed out that this approach may not be suitable for long-term serial studies because film processing techniques change over time.

Although theoretically easy, it is difficult to process X-ray films consistently to a good standard quality. Also, since skilled radiographers are rare, special training programmes may prove useful in reducing variability in classification.

Medical and occupational history and physical examination

A medical history with special emphasis on past and present occupations and their relationship with the symptoms being examined is essential for the purposes of differential diagnosis. From the medical/occupational history it is also possible to estimate the time that has elapsed between exposure and the onset of symptoms and hence to assess the severity of the disease. Many modifications of the British Medical Research Council (MRC) questionnaire for individual respiratory occupational diseases are available (see, for example, Annex 1). However, for best results they must be used in the local vernacular. An accurate smoking history should always be taken.

---

[1] *Guidelines for the use of ILO International Classification of Radiographs of Pneumoconioses. Revised edition 1980.* Geneva, International Labour Office, 1980 (Occupational Safety and Health Series, 22 (rev. 80)).

A physical examination is also essential. However, it should be stated that an occupational and medical history (taken with the help of MRC-type questionnaires) and lung function tests give a more accurate assessment of the severity of disease and disability than does a physical examination.

Lung function tests

Fortunately, the simplest (and cheapest) tests have proved to be reliable enough for epidemiological work and screening programmes. Because of local variations in the characteristics of different populations and of the fact that workforces are usually biased (healthy) samples of the general population, published "normal" values for lung function tests have limited use; however, values corrected for height, age, sex, and smoking habits can be used. Whenever possible, standard values and correction factors should be developed at each factory by including workers with negligible, low, moderate, and high levels of exposure.

(1) Spirometry

Easy to use, robust, relatively cheap, dry-bellow spirometers are available. They can be used to perform various tests, but the forced expiratory volume in one second ($FEV_{1.0}$) and forced vital capacity (FVC) are most useful and repeatable. Both readings can be made from the same expiratory effort. The final reading in both cases is the mean of 3 breaths, which are preceded by two practice breaths. In both cases, the tests should be repeated if the variation between the 3 breaths is over 5%. $FEV_{1.0}$ is repeatable to within 5%, FVC is slightly less constant, especially in women. All results should be corrected for age, height, and especially smoking habit.

It should be noted that smoking lowers $FEV_{1.0}$ and FVC values more than any occupational health hazard. Thus, the significance of these tests in smokers should be judged with caution.

Other tests possible with spirometry include, for example, measurements of small airway function, airway resistance, compliance, and lung volume. These tests may be useful in the differential diagnosis of certain types of exposure or in complicated individual cases.

(2) Peak-flow rate measurements

Peak-flow rate (PFR) is the maximum rate of expiratory flow during a forced exhalation. It is a useful substitute for the $FEV_{1.0}$ test when frequent serial readings are required. The correlation between peak-flow measurements and $FEV_{1.0}$ values is very high. However corrections for height, age, and smoking habit are necessary. The equipment for this test is portable and very cheap. Although this test is less informative than $FEV_{1.0}$ and FVC measurements for long-term epidemiological purposes, the chief value of PFR is in the detection and measurement of changes in airway function during the workshift and during the night and the weekend (e.g., in screening for byssinosis and occupational asthma).

The mean of three readings after two practice breaths is calculated. Since the error associated with this method is less than 5%, a fall of greater than 15% during a workshift is considered clinically significant in individual cases; a fall of more than 5% in the mean value is significant in groups.

(3) Gas transfer measurements

These require more expensive equipment and more worker cooperation than the simple spirometric and PFR measurements. However, they are the best available indicators of alveolar disease. The error between individual measurements is relatively high (up to 15%) and the normal range (either published or within test populations) is wide. Serial values are also affected by intercurrent illnesses, and by changes in airways.

The test for the measurement of gas transfer is usually performed on a single breath using 0.25–0.30% carbon monoxide and 2–12% helium and it includes a measurement of the lung volume. It should be pointed out here that it may not be possible to carry out this test in workers who, owing to their disability, cannot hold their breath for the time required for making the measurement. The result should be corrected for age, height, and smoking habit. Other tests of alveolar function (such as tests of mixing, ventilation test, arterial blood gas measurements, and exercise tests) have not proved useful in the early detection of occupational disease in groups of workers, but may be useful in the investigation of complicated individual cases.

Application and usefulness of lung function tests

The most informative diagnostic procedure is to combine medical and occupational history (especially one taken with the help of a well designed questionnaire) with a physical examination. Radiology is essential in diagnosing pneumoconioses due to mineral dusts.

Lung function tests are of particular value in diagnosing bronchial disorders. $FEV_{1.0}$, FVC, and PFR are the most useful tests in field conditions. However, nowadays it is possible to adapt more complex tests to field conditions (e.g., by designing a special testing van), particularly for epidemiological studies.

CHAPTER 31

The nervous system

Function

The peripheral nerves are composed mainly of sensory (afferent) and motor (efferent) fibres. These carry:

(a) the sensory mechanoreceptive,[1] thermoreceptive, and pain impulses originating in the specific receptors to the somatesthetic area in the cerebral cortex via the spinal cord and brain stem sensory tracts;

(b) the motor impulses from the spinal cord to the effectors—i.e., the skeletal muscles.

The *cerebral cortex* is a highly specialized area of the brain where impulses conveyed by the sensory afferent nerves (responsible for general, visual, auditory, and gustatory sensation) and the efferent motor nerves (responsible for the contraction of skeletal muscles) are integrated. The remainder of the cortex falls under the general heading of association cortex, which controls the complex behavioural and intellectual functions.

The main portion of the *extrapyramidal system* is represented by the basal ganglia, the function of which is to control muscle movements, muscular tonus, gait, and facial expression. The *cerebellum* is essentially a motor part of the brain. It is responsible for the maintenance of equilibrium and coordination of muscle action, and it contributes to the synergy of muscular action.

Pathophysiological mechanisms

Metabolic changes in nervous tissue due to either the direct action of undesirable chemicals or the impairment of oxygen supply (ischaemic vascular changes) seem to be the main factors responsible for the development of neuropathy. It has been suggested that a number of chemically unrelated industrial agents, such as carbon disulfide and acrylamide, act by interfering with glycolytic enzymes containing sulfhydryl groups, namely glyceraldehyde-3-phosphate dehydrogenase and phosphofructokinase.

---

[1] The mechanoreceptors are receptors that are excited by mechanical pressures or distortions, such as touch, pressure, movement (kinaesthesia), or changes in posture.

Methyl-n-butyl ketone has been shown to reduce adenosine triphosphate (ATP) in nerve tissues. The resultant lack of energy causes disruption of energy-demanding processes, such as the axonal transport and the repolarization of the nerve fibre, both of which are necessary for trophic influxes and impulse transmission.

Organophosphorus compounds act by inhibiting cholinesterase activity. Direct transfer of physical energy to nervous tissues is supposed to be a contributing factor in vibration-related neuropathies. Segmental demyelination (loss of the myelin sheath involving limited internodal areas, with preservation of the axon) and axonal degeneration are the histological features of polyneuropathy. The degeneration of the axon results in a more severe form of neuropathy, which often begins in the more distal parts of the nerves, slowly reaching the proximal segments; it is also called distal axonopathy.

Common occupational neurological disorders and differential diagnosis

Agents causing occupational neurological disorders affect both central and peripheral nervous systems. At the present time, there appears to be some disagreement between experts as to which of the two systems is more frequently affected. This is probably due to differences in the criteria and diagnostic procedures employed in the investigations as well as to the different types and levels of exposure studied. The protection offered by the blood–brain barrier against the penetration of toxic substances into the brain may explain in part the more frequent damage to peripheral nerves reported by some authors.

Organic solvents and asphyxiants cause predominantly central nervous system damage, which ranges from mild disturbances of consciousness to coma and which may be permanent. Table 5 summarizes common occupational neurological disorders.

Uncontrolled long- or medium-term exposure to neurotoxic substances or physical agents may result in nerve fibre impairment, causing the clinical picture of polyneuropathy. However, under the present-day environmental conditions in industry and agriculture in industrialized countries, severe poisonings are becoming less frequent, though epidemic outbreaks may still occur (for example, neuropathies from heavy accidental exposure to methyl n-butyl ketone and acrylamide or industrial adhesives). On the other hand, minor subclinical cases are increasingly observed, particularly in exposure to carbon disulfide and organic solvents. However, the situation is probably different and more serious in developing countries.

An important clinical feature of neuropathies caused by toxic agents is the simultaneous and symmetrical involvement of many nerves. This may sometimes help in distinguishing occupation-related disorders from other peripheral neuropathies, such as radiculopathies and mononeuropathies due to other causes (trauma, collagen vascular

Table 5. Common occupational neurological disorders and their causes

Disorder	Main causes
Peripheral neuropathy	
Polyneuropathy (distal, symmetrical)	A number of chemicals, such as lead, arsenic, trichloroethylene, methyl n-butyl ketone, carbon disulfide, n-hexane, acrylamide, o-cresyl phosphate, etc.
Mononeuropathy	Vibration
Psycho-organic disease (organic brain syndrome)	Various aliphatic and aromatic hydrocarbons, carbon disulfide, mercury, lead
Encephalopathy (similar to vascular encephalopathy)	Carbon disulfide, lead
Extrapyramidal disorders	Manganese, carbon disulfide, mercury
Cerebellar disorders	Mercury

disease, etc). The onset of occupational neurological disorders is usually subacute. However, occasionally it may be acute, and in such instances it is necessary to differentiate toxic polyneuropathy from acute infective polyneuritis (Guillain-Barré syndrome). Long-standing paraesthesias (tingling, pins and needles, coldness, and cramp-like pain in the calves) may for years precede the appearance of clear-cut clinical symptoms.

In occupational neurological disorders a sensorimotor, distal, non-lateral neuropathy is the typical pattern, with flaccid muscular weakness in the distal muscles and a typical stocking/glove sensory loss; the sense of position is occasionally altered with consequent ataxia. Motor impairment is generally prominent in the distal muscles of the limbs and, in severe cases, drop foot and drop wrist (lead poisoning) are present, the former causing a steppage gait. Proximal muscles are rarely affected. However, some authors have observed motor impairment in proximal muscles of the limbs in neuropathy due to leather glues. Deep tendon reflexes are diminished or lost in the early stages, and the loss of Achilles tendon reflex precedes the loss of patellar reflex. The cerebrospinal fluid is generally normal. Apparently, sometimes purely motor or sensory neuropathies also occur. However, neurophysiological testing has shown that both sensory and motor fibres are affected. The rate of progression of the condition varies greatly, but the prognosis is usually good if the subject is removed from exposure. Motor sequelae may be present and so may persisting neurophysiological abnormalities. The cranial nerves are affected less often than other nerves. However, there are reports of damage to the optic nerve (from methanol, carbon disulfide) and to the acoustic nerve (from trichloroethylene).

The symptoms of psycho-organic disease (organic brain syndrome) vary considerably and include: depression, erethism, low vigilance and attention, memory impairment, and reduction of mental efficiency. This syndrome is generally rather uniform in different types of exposure. However, psychomotor activation may predominate in some exposures (e.g., to mercury), while depression is more frequently seen in subjects exposed to organic solvents and carbon disulfide.

Tests

Neurological examination

The neurological examination must include an accurate occupational and medical history with regard to nervous function, the following must be evaluated: mental status, cranial nerves, motor and sensory systems, reflexes, coordination, gait, and station. An evaluation of the autonomic nervous system (pupillary light reflex and the lacrimal, salivary and digestive, and urinary and sexual functions) must be carried out. It is recommended that deep tendon reflexes and muscular strength be carefully examined and evaluated.

Measurement of vibration sensitivity

The measurement of vibration sensitivity provides information on the condition of the nerve fibres carrying deep sensation, and is considered an excellent tool for the assessment of sensory impairment. The test involves the application of a tuning fork (range 128–256 Hz) to a bony eminence. More recently, there has been a tendency to quantify vibration sensitivity by electromagnetic or electrically produced vibrations.

Neurophysiological tests

Electromyography and nerve conduction tests (electroneurography) are the two main neurophysiological investigations employed; they can not only confirm the diagnosis of manifest neuropathy, but can also detect subclinical cases.

Electromyography can help detect denervation of muscle fibres resulting from axonal or wallerian degeneration. Moreover, it can demonstrate electric potentials in the resting muscle (fibrillation, positive sharp waves), reduced recruitment of motor units during muscular contraction (intermediate or single units pattern), and variation in the motor unit parameters (increased duration and amplitude in long-standing conditions) and in morphology (increased polyphasic potentials).

Electroneurography permits the measurement of the conduction velocity of the impulses of both motor and sensory fibres. The median, ulnar, and peroneal nerves are usually studied. In general, the slowing of motor and sensory conduction velocities is considered a sensitive sign of incipient neuropathy from segmental demyelination or of incomplete recovery when it persists after the clinical findings have completely regressed. If the technical conditions of the examination are standardized, the values of motor and sensory conduction velocity are sufficiently reproducible. Skin temperature can affect nerve conduction and should be controlled. A number of interfering factors should also be carefully evaluated as a source of variability: age, alcohol consumption, long-term use of therapeutic drugs, diabetes, cervical or lumbar spondylosis, etc. If these factors are properly taken into account and if electroneurography is performed at regular intervals in high-risk groups, the conduction velocity test can be considered a useful and non-invasive method for the early detection of neuropathies and their prevention. The periodicity of the examination depends to a large extent on the qualitative and quantitative characteristics of exposure. Electromyography also provides important information on the condition of the nerve fibre axons, but it is doubtful whether it can be recommended as a screening method since it is partially invasive, requiring the insertion of needles into the muscles.

Electroencephalography

Electroencephalography cannot be recommended as a test for the early detection of functional impairment of the central nervous system. The same is true for new techniques such as brain-evoked potentials and electroencephalographic frequency analysis. Although these two methods are valid in the differential diagnosis of early central nervous system impairment, they are rather complicated and therefore cannot as yet be recommended for screening purposes.

Psychological tests

High-risk workers exposed to neurotoxic substances should undergo periodic psychological examinations in order to prevent the occurrence of irreversible deterioration of higher nervous system functions. If possible, a baseline profile should be obtained prior to exposure for use as reference for subsequent examinations. The tests for baseline profile and later control should include:

—a measure of intellectual dynamism (e.g., Raven PM38 test)
—a test of memory, including mechanical, visual, and logical components (e.g., Wechsler memory tests);
—a personality screening to show the possible existence of neurotic-like personality traits; and
—reaction times.

Special attention should be paid to subjective reports of emotional and/or mental discomfort. These feelings are often the only early evidence of impairment of higher nervous functions. If the symptoms suggest a more severe involvement of the central nervous system, a thorough psychodiagnostic investigation should be carried out in order to explore the integrity of the central nervous system functions, including: mental dynamism in relation to cultural intellectual capacity; short and delayed memory; capacity of retention, storage and reproduction of information; psychomotor abilities; and personality alterations affecting the individual and the social sphere of existence.

Psychological tests are considered to be sensitive indicators of early mental and emotional disorders. However, it is often difficult to differentiate functional psychogenic impairments from organic deterioration processes. In this regard, individual baseline profiles can of course be of substantial help in the diagnosis. But when a baseline profile is not available, the following points should be considered in the diagnosis:

—functional impairments are less specific than signs of organic deterioration processes;
—functional impairments have a more profound effect on the personality than on mental functions;
—functional impairments vary with time and are reversible.

Considering the limited facilities available in most countries for thorough psychological examinations, it is difficult to recommend a general time interval applicable to all situations. However, a reasonable interval would probably be two years.

Whenever possible, subjects affected by emotional or mental conditions should not be employed in occupations involving exposure to neurotoxic agents.

CHAPTER 32

Blood and the blood-forming system

Function

The two main functions of blood are:
—to transport oxygen (in haemoglobin) and carbon dioxide to and from the tissues, respectively;
—to transport products of anabolism and catabolism, hormones, antibodies, enzymes, minerals, etc.

Blood cells are almost entirely produced in the bone marrow, with a minor part of the lymphocytes being produced in the lymphopoietic tissue.

Pathophysiological mechanisms

The most common blood-related affection of occupational origin is the decrease in the number of blood elements. There are two main etiologies: (a) decreased production of blood cells in the bone marrow (central cytopenia); and (b) increased destruction of blood cells in peripheral blood (peripheral cytopenia). The former is caused by damage to the bone marrow by toxic substances and ionizing radiation, and rarely, by immunological mechanisms. Bone marrow damage is frequently accompanied by disturbances in haemoglobin synthesis. Haemolytic anaemias may be caused by direct toxic damage to the erythrocyte membrane, formation of intraerythrocytic Heinz bodies (resulting from oxidative injury to and precipitation of haemoglobin), or by immunological mechanism. Peripheral leukopenia and thrombocytopenia are as a rule of immunological etiology.

Other frequent affections related to changes in haemoglobin include, for example, carboxyhaemoglobinaemia (reversible replacement of oxygen by carbon monoxide) and methaemoglobinaemia (reversible oxidation of the Fe^{2+} in haeme into Fe^{3+}), both of which result in the impairment of oxygen transport.

Leukaemias are neoplastic diseases, supposingly resulting from changes in the genetic material of haematopoietic precursor cells. Ionizing radiation and benzene have leukaemogenic properties.

Haemorrhagic diatheses (increased tendency to bleed) result from decreased number or dysfunction of thrombocytes, defects of coagulation factors in the blood plasma, or capillary wall disorders.

Common disorders and differential diagnosis

The main haematological disorders are summarized in Table 6. Slight shifts in haematological parameters have been reported as a result of exposure to many chemical and physical factors. However, such changes have no proven clinical significance.

The differential diagnosis of haematological disorders does not usually present any major problems in acute poisonings (haemolysis, leukocytosis, methaemoglobinaemia). Thus, only the problems associated with long-term exposures are discussed below.

Heinz bodies and methaemoglobin are found mainly in poisonings by aromatic, amino, and nitro compounds (like aniline, nitrobenzene, nitric acid esters, nitroglycols, etc.). They may also appear during treatment with antimalarial and other drugs in susceptible individuals, e.g., in those suffering from erythrocytic enzymopenias (e.g., glucose-6-phosphate dehydrogenase deficiency) or haemoglobinopathies (e.g., thalassaemia). If methaemoglobinaemia and Heinz bodies appear repeatedly in a worker exposed to low concentrations of the above-mentioned chemicals, tests for possible hypersensitivity should be

Table 6.   Main haematological disorders and their causes

Disorder	Main causes
Anaemia	
Haemolytic	Arsine (direct haemolysis); aromatic amino and nitro compounds (haemolysis due to the formation of Heinz bodies); immunological changes
Dyshaematopoietic	Lead
Aplastic	Benzene, trinitrotoluene, ionizing radiation
Secondary	Bleeding, renal failure, etc.
Polycythaemia	Respiratory insufficiency in chronic pneumopathies (pneumoconioses); toxic chemicals (cobalt, carbon monoxide, manganese); haemoconcentration (dehydration in acute poisoning)
Leukopenia, thrombocytopenia	
Central	Bone marrow suppression; benzene; trinitrotoluene; ionizing radiation
Peripheral	Immunological changes
Leukocytosis	Acute poisonings (early phases); infectious diseases
Leukaemia	Benzene; ionizing radiation
Haemorrhagic diathesis	Radiation; benzene; uraemia
Secondary	Liver failure
Methaemoglobinaemia	Aromatic amino and nitro compounds; esters of nitric acid

performed. In countries where there is a high prevalence of erythrocytic enzymopenias or haemoglobinopathies, a check for hypersensitivity at the pre-employment health examination is recommended.

In assessing the occupational origin of *bone marrow suppression*, both the clinical course of the disease and the level of exposure to the suspected health hazard should be considered. Since idiopathic or drug-induced bone marrow hypoplasias or aplasias also occur in the general population, an occupational etiology should be suspected only when there is evidence of high-level occupational exposure to a known bone-marrow depressant.

Peripheral leukopenia and thrombocytopenia are mainly of immunological etiology. They may be caused by a great number of substances, particularly drugs, the best known of which is aminophenazone (agranulocytosis). Among the occupational agents, pesticides are the main suspects. However, it should be pointed out that almost all chemicals found in the working environment have been associated with cytopenia. The lack of adequate laboratory methods makes the assessment of immunological mechanisms in cytopenias difficult. A causal relationship can be suspected if cytopenia develops on several successive occasions after exposure to a chemical substance. The causality is confirmed only when cytopenia appears regularly after each exposure or if corresponding antibodies are found *in vitro*.

Benzene and ionizing radiation have been shown to be *leukaemogenic*. Epidemiological data show increased incidence of acute nonlymphocytic leukaemias and chronic granulocytic leukaemias following exposure to benzene and radiation; the former is also known to cause erythroleukaemias. Some authors claim that benzene and ionizing radiation also induce other haemoblastoses, but convincing evidence has not been given.

Haemorrhagic diathesis may occur in acute disease following irradiation exposure, chronic benzene poisoning, thrombocytopenia, thromboasthenia, diseases of capillary walls, and possibly, also in disorders of plasmatic coagulation factors. Secondary haemocoagulation disturbances may develop in severe liver and renal insufficiencies, including those of occupational origin.

Tests

Methods of examination and normal values

Haematological methods have been largely standardized by WHO.[1] The normal values are given in Table 7.

---

[1] *Manual of basic techniques for a health laboratory.* Geneva, World Health Organization, 1980.

Table 7. Normal range of haematological values

Erythrocyte number concentration (cells $\times 10^{12}$ per litre)	men women	4.5–5.5 4.0–5.0
Haemoglobin (Fe) concentration (mmol) per litre	men women	8.1–11.2 7.1–10.2
Erythrocyte volume fraction	men women	0.40–0.50 0.37–0.43
Leukocyte number concentration (cells $\times 10^9$ per litre)		4–10
Leukocyte type number fraction: neutrophils eosinophils basophils lymphocytes monocytes		0.55–0.65 0.02–0.04 0–0.01 0.25–0.35 0.03–0.06
Reticulocyte number concentration (cells $\times 10^9$ per litre)		8–110
Thrombocyte number concentration (number $\times 10^9$ per litre)		about 300 000
Bleeding time (min)		1–5
Coagulation time (min)		5–12

Source: Manual of basic techniques for a health laboratory. Geneva, World Health Organization, 1980.

Evaluation of results

Whereas normal values for erythrocyte count and haemoglobin concentration remain rather stable (variations at repeated examinations should not exceed $\pm 10\%$), the leukocyte count may show considerable variation. Intra-individual variations are quite common, and are triggered by external factors or unknown reasons. Thus, single values may occasionally exceed normal limits. Values lower than 4×10^9 are also found in a small percentage of healthy individuals. Such low values do not represent any health impairment if they are not accompanied by pathological morphological changes in blood cells, or if they have not declined from previously higher values. In occupational medicine, any rational evaluation of blood count requires comparison with previous (preplacement) values.

Usefulness of haematological tests

In screening workers for early signs of anaemias, it is sufficient to measure the haemoglobin concentration only. If the result is outside the normal range then a complete haematological examination (blood count, blood film) should be done.

In occupations involving exposure to agents known to affect the blood-forming tissues (e.g., benzene, trinitrotoluene, ionizing radiation), the preplacement examination should include a full blood count and the determination of haemoglobin concentration. This examination should be repeated at intervals depending on the level of exposure. The detection of early signs of depression of blood elements is possible only if a baseline measurement is available.

More complicated methods, such as bone marrow aspiration, measurement of coagulation factors, etc. may be necessary for differential diagnosis in complicated cases. However, they have no use in regular periodic examinations.

CHAPTER 33

The digestive system—gastrointestinal tract and liver

Functions

The ingested food and other materials (ingested accidentally or intentionally) are digested and absorbed in the gastrointestinal tract. Most of the ingested food is first broken down into absorbable chemical substances through the action of enzymes in saliva and in gastric, pancreatic, and intestinal juices. Hydrochloric acid and bile juice (which is secreted by the liver) are other important agents in the process of digestion.

The liver is essential to life. Its numerous functions include: storage and filtration of blood; secretion of bile; metabolism of organic substances (biotransformation); excretion of bilirubin and other substances formed elsewhere in the body; and protein synthesis.

In occupational exposure, the gastrointestinal tract is a major route of entry into the body of toxic substances, particularly solid toxic substances. Also, when airborne particulate matter is cleared from the lungs and deposited at the nasopharynx, the particles may be swallowed and absorbed in the gastrointestinal tract.

Pathophysiological mechanisms

A large number of chemicals are corrosive and their ingestion causes severe damage to the gastrointestinal tract, irrespective of any systemic action. Even those normally not considered to be corrosive (e.g., most solvents) are highly irritant to the tissues and cause vomiting, pain, and diarrhoea. Absorption of such substances, almost certainly follows and may cause systemic poisoning.

In long-term exposure, few chemicals exert their main toxic action on the gastrointestinal tract, though poisonings by many substances may be accompanied by symptoms or signs of gastrointestinal involvement.

The liver is the target organ for the toxic effects of many chemicals. It is also the major site for their biotransformation. The mechanisms involved in liver damage by most substances are still unknown. It is established that mercury and arsenic combine with enzymes containing sulfhydryl groups and thus interfere with hepatic metabolic functions.

225

A number of substances including haloalkanes and haloalkenes may be activated by the mixed-function oxidase enzymes of the liver into reactive, but unstable, components (such as the radical CCl_3^- derived from carbon tetrachloride and the epoxides formed from halothanes and aromatic agents); these components may, in turn, "attack" cellular constituents or initiate destructive processes such as lipid peroxidation.

Toxic liver injury usually takes the form of periportal or centrilobular necrosis of the cells, and may be extensive in cases of high exposure. Following chronic injury, the damaged tissue becomes fibrous, and this process can progress to cirrhosis. Either of these can result in acute or progressive liver failure.

Common disorders and differential diagnosis

Occupational conditions directly affecting the digestive tract

Long-term exposure to fumes of nitric, sulfuric, and hydrochloric acids may cause erosion of the upper and lower incisors, typically affecting the incisal edges and extending to the labial surfaces. The enamel may be destroyed, rendering the dentin exposed to attack and causing brown or black discoloration of the teeth. The condition is usually painless but disfiguring. With periodic dental examinations it may be possible to detect the condition at an early stage. Protective masks may have some value, but technical measures to control the release of acid fumes are the only effective means of prevention.

Yellow phosphorus causes necrosis of the bone of the jaw, the early stages of which are characterized by dental pain and inflammation of the gum.

Conditions causing symptoms or signs related to the digestive tract

Many substances may cause symptoms and signs involving the gastrointestinal system, including those whose primary targets for toxic action are other organs (see Table 8). Occasionally, the signs and symptoms are specific for certain types of exposure. For example, a blue line may be observed on the gum margins of workers exposed to lead, indicating lead absorption, but not necessarily lead poisoning. Similarly swelling and bleeding of the gums is an early sign of mercury poisoning.

Liver damage

(1) Toxic hepatitis

A list of chemical substances reported to have caused toxic liver damage in occupational exposure is given in Table 9.

Table 8. Digestive tract symptoms and their main causes

Effect	Main causes
Gingivitis, glossitis, stomatitis	Lead (blue line), mercury (gingivitis, blue/brown line)
Oesophageal bleeding from varices resulting from liver cirrhosis	Vinyl chloride and other liver toxins
Gastritis	Cadmium and its salts, carbon disulfide, chloronaphthalenes, chromium and its compounds
Abdominal pain	Arsine, bromochloromethane, lead (colic), phosphine, tetrabromoethane
Diarrhoea or constipation	Lead (chronic constipation), mercury (diarrhoea)

Table 9. Substances reported to have caused toxic liver injury in occupational exposure

Metals	Halogenated compounds	Other substances
Arsenic	Carbon tetrachloride	Alcohols (methyl, ethyl, propyl, etc.)
Antimony	Chloroform	Carbon disulfide
Mercury	Chloronaphthalenes	Dimethyl nitrosamine
Phosphorus	Dibromochloropropane	Dioxane
Selenium	1,2-dichloroethane	Epichlorohydrin
	Ethylene dibromide	Kepone
	Ethylene dichloride	Methylene dianiline
	Methyl bromide	Naphthalene
	Methyl chloride	Naphthol
	Tetrabromoethane	Nitrobenzene
	Tetrachloroethane	Pyrogallol
	Trichloroethane	Trinitrotoluene
	Trichloroethylene	Polychlorinated biphenyls
	Tetrachloroethylene	Polybrominated biphenyls

The hepatotoxic effects of carbon tetrachloride, chloroform, methyl bromide, tetrachloroethane, arsenic, and yellow phosphorus, even in relatively small doses, are well proven. Other chemicals mentioned above have been reported to cause serious acute poisoning and liver damage following very high exposure.

(2) Occupational infections of the liver

Leptospirosis (Weil's disease) is a liver infection caused by *Leptospira interrogans* or other members of the genus *Leptospira* of which the natural hosts are rodents (e.g., mice, rats). Persons working in rat-infested surroundings (e.g., sewer workers, fish cleaners, veterinarians, farmers, dock workers, and animal breeders) are at risk of contracting this disease.

Viral hepatitis is an acute generalized infection causing widespread damage, including necrosis of liver cells. The clinical picture can range from mild gastrointestinal symptoms through acute icteric illness to acute fulminant hepatitis. Type B infections are generally more severe than Type A infections, and may also progress more frequently to chronic liver disease.

(3) Occupational tumour of the liver

So far, the only primary liver tumour that has been clearly shown to be associated with occupational exposure is the haemangiosarcoma in workers exposed to vinyl chloride monomer. The highest incidence of this tumour is found in workers heavily exposed to unreacted monomer during the manual cleaning of the autoclaves used for polymerization in the manufacture of polyvinyl chloride. No evidence of a health hazard has been found among workers engaged in the moulding or processing of polyvinyl chloride in the manufacture of plastic products.

Some of the workers shown to have developed haemangiosarcomas of the liver following heavy exposure to vinyl chloride also had nonspecific periportal fibrosis resembling primary biliary cirrhosis. It has been suggested that angiosarcomata may develop in these chronically injured tissues (see also the section on vinyl chloride in Chapter 17):

Tests

Medical examination

Routine medical examinations for gastrointestinal symptoms are useful only when there is clear evidence that the working population in question is regularly exposed to a toxic substance known to cause such effects, e.g., yellow phosphorus and hepatotoxic agents.

A medical history (including that of alcohol consumption) and a physical examination, with special attention to liver palpation and urinalysis (urobilinogen and bile pigments), are essential. The most sensitive test of liver cell damage is the measurement of serum activity of the enzymes released fom hepatocytes.

Laboratory tests

Hepatocytes contain many enzymes that may be released into the blood if the cell membranes become damaged. The two most important enzymes are: aspartate aminotransferase (E.C.2.6.1.1) (alternative name: glutamic oxaloacetic transaminase) and alanine aminotransferase (E.C.2.6.1.2) (alternative name: glutamic pyruvic transaminase). The alkaline phosphatase (E.C.3.1.3.1) level in the blood may increase when hepatocytes are killed rather than damaged, as may happen in cholestasis (obstruction of biliary pathways). Gamma-glutamyl transferase (E.C.2.3.2.2) is a microsomal enzyme which may be elevated in many liver diseases and in response to hepatotoxins that induce the release of hepatic enzymes (including ethanol). The levels of lactate dehydrogenase (E.C.1.1.1.27) or, more specifically, L-iditol dehydrogenase (E.C.1.1.1.14) also rise as a result of hepatocellular damage, and their measurements are frequently used as indices of such damage.

Serum bilirubin gives an accurate measure of the extent of jaundice, and repeated estimations may be useful in following the progress of parenchymal liver disease.

In practice, the estimation of the activity of one of the transferases and bilirubin concentration provide all the information needed in screening for toxic and viral hepatitis. For differential diagnosis, however, a full range of tests may be necessary.

In liver injury due to vinyl chloride, the biochemical tests of hepatic function are of limited value in detecting slight hepatic damage, and the significance of marginally abnormal test results is difficult to determine. A number of more sophisticated procedures have been proposed for the early detection of vinyl chloride hepatic damage, such as ultrasonography of the liver, microvascular skin capillary assessment, urinary analysis of glucosaminoglycan excretion, and radionucleotide ([99]S) liver scanning. However, it should be noted that none of these tests provides sufficient sensitivity or specificity to warrant its use in screening for subclinical asymptomatic hepatic injury in workers exposed to hepatotoxic chemicals.

At present, therefore, the value of screening procedures in the early detection of vinyl chloride liver disease is limited. Preplacement screening for the detection of subjects with chronic liver disease or persistent biochemical abnormalities has some value; therefore relevant tests should be performed before engaging new workers for work involving exposure to vinyl chloride monomer.

Application and usefulness

The biochemical tests mentioned above as well the many others available were developed mainly for the purposes of differential diagnosis and to confirm the clinical diagnosis in overtly ill patients.

They are of far less value in detecting slight or early damage. It is probably not worth while to undertake continuous screening of clinically healthy workers by means of these tests because the results are likely to be confusing and impossible to interpret rather than helpful.

CHAPTER 34

The urinary system

Functions

The kidneys help to ensure the efficient functioning of body cells through a number of mechanisms: (a) regulation of the extracellular fluid volume; (b) control of electrolytes and acid–base balance; (c) excretion of toxic and waste products; and (d) conservation of essential substances. In addition, the kidneys have an endocrine function (production of haemopoietin, response to aldosterone, antidiuretic and parathyroid hormones).

Pathophysiological mechanisms

Different nephrotoxic agents act at different sites on the tubular epithelium. For example, arsine, cadmium, lead, and mercury act on the proximal straight tubule, and paraquat and phosphorus act on the proximal convoluted, proximal straight, and distal convoluted tubules. The extent of the damage depends on the level of exposure.

In occupational exposure, glomerular damage is less frequent, and acute poisonings are often associated with severe shock. Clinically, the sequence of shock oliguria, diuresis, and post-diuretic phase follows a similar course to that of acute tubular necrosis, except that oliguria is usually more prolonged.

In chronic urinary tract disturbances, it is possible to detect altered biological functions before the appearance of subjective symptoms or clinical signs. An early sign of renal damage (glomerular or tubular) induced by many nephrotoxic chemicals is increased urinary excretion of proteins. Normally, the amount of proteins excreted in the urine does not exceed 250 mg per day. These proteins originate from the urogenital tract (approximately 50%) and the plasma. Proteins cross the glomerular filter in proportion to their molecular dimension: those with a molecular mass below 40 000 pass easily through the glomerular filter, whereas proteins with a molecular mass above 40 000 are more effectively retained. The filtered proteins are reabsorbed by the proximal tubular cells of the kidney.

In glomerular damage, the glomerular permeability is usually increased and therefore larger quantities of high-molecular-mass proteins enter the glomerular filtrate and ultimately appear in the

231

urine. The urinary concentration of low-molecular-mass proteins is not increased since the reabsorption process in the tubule is normal.

When proteinuria is a consequence of tubular dysfunction, the amount of protein filtered through the glomeruli is not increased, but the low- and the high-molecular-mass proteins, which are normally filtered, appear in larger quantities in the final urine, because the tubular reabsorption is incomplete. However, the urinary concentration of low-molecular-mass proteins is proportionally more increased than that of high-molecular-mass proteins. In tubular proteinuria, protein loss is usually less than 2 g/24 h. When both sites—the glomeruli and the tubules—are damaged, the proteinuria consists of a mixture of low- and high-molecular-mass proteins.

Common disorders and differential diagnosis

Effects on the kidney

Acute effects include:
—acute tubular necrosis (mercury, several halogenated aliphatic hydrocarbons)
—indirect toxic effects of haemolytic poisons (e.g., arsine)
Chronic effects include:
—glomerular and/or tubular dysfunction (lead, cadmium, mercury)
—renal tumour (coke-oven emissions)

Effect on the urinary tract

Effects on the urinary tract include:
—neurogenic cystitis (dimethyl aminopropionitrite)
—bladder tumour (several aromatic amines, such as benzidine and β-naphthylamine)

Whereas in acute poisonings the etiology is usually immediately obvious the attribution of occupational etiology to chronic urinary tract impairment is more equivocal, and is based on evidence of preceding exposure and of changes typical of the suspected causal agent.

Tests

The detection of toxic effects of industrial chemicals on the urinary system involves: (*a*) a detailed investigation of the individual's subjective symptoms possibly related to renal and urinary tract disturbances (dysuria, pollakiuria, etc.); (*b*) a complete medical examination (including in some cases prostate palpation); and (*c*) the performance of appropriate biological analyses.

The laboratory tests can be divided in two groups: (*a*) Screening tests, suitable for the periodic medical surveillance in industry;

and (*b*) functional tests, which are usually performed only when the screening tests are abnormal or when the symptoms are specific enough to suspect the presence of a renal disease.

Screening tests

Screening tests may be performed on either urine or blood. It should be stressed that for any of these tests a single determination may be misleading. Repeated determinations are necessary in order to confirm the presence of a renal function change.

(1) *Urine analyses*

Preferably, the urine analyses should be carried out on a 24-hour urine sample. Unfortunately, however, a complete 24-hour urine collection is extremely difficult to obtain. Even the analysis of a morning specimen is not always feasible, and frequently, in occupational medical practice, the analyses have to be performed on spot specimens. It is therefore important to evaluate the degree of urine dilution (specific gravity, creatinine concentration, osmolality) because analyses performed on very dilute urine specimens are not reliable and may give false negative results).

(*a*) *Appearance of urine.* The appearance provides very limited information, but since it is so simple to perform it should never be neglected.

(*b*) *Reagent strip for protein and glucose.* Normally, the amount of protein excreted in urine does not exceed 250 mg per day. Screening tests using a reagent strip for the detection of free aminogroups are more sensitive to albumin than to globulin. They will detect albumin concentrations ranging from 50 to 300 mg/litre. False positive results may be obtained with alkaline urine and quarternary ammonium compounds.

Screening tests based on reagent strips will not detect an increased urinary excretion of low-molecular-mass proteins and they are too coarse for the detection of proteinuria of less than 0.5 g/day, as found in the early stage of renal tubular dysfunction or in the relatively inactive phase of glomerular disease. For such purposes, more sensitive, quantitative methods must be used (see below). Although glucose is also frequently excreted in kidney damage, the determination of glucosuria cannot be used as renal screening test.

(*c*) *Quantitative determination of total protein in urine.* The detection of a slightly increased total proteinuria (< 0.5 g/24 h) requires the use of a quantitative method (e.g., the biuret method). To be of significance, this test should be carried out on urine collected during a well defined time interval (24 hour or less) and the results should be confirmed by repeated measurements. However, in the early stages of metal-induced renal dysfunction, it is usual to find significantly increased urinary excretion of specific proteins (e.g., retinol-binding protein or

β_2-microglobulin in workers exposed to cadmium) without significant change in total protein excretion.

(*d*) *Quantitative determination of specific proteins in urine.* Sensitive immunochemical methods are now available for the quantitative analysis of specific proteins in urine. The determination of at least one low-molecular-mass protein (e.g., either retinol-binding protein or β_2-microglobulin) and one high-molecular-mass protein (e.g., albumin) should be included in the surveillance programme of workers exposed to cadmium and possibly other nephrotoxic metals. It should be noted that, for the determination of some proteins (e.g., β_2-microglobulin), the control of the urinary pH is important.

(*e*) *Electrophoretic characterization of proteinuria.* The electrophoretic or immunoelectrophoretic separation of urinary proteins can also be used to classify the proteinuria in three categories: glomerular, tubular, or mixed proteinuria. For this test, the urine sample has to be concentrated.

(*f*) *Examination of urine sediment.* This analysis is useful in diagnosing renal parenchymal damage (e.g., presence of cell cylinders) and confirming the presence of haematuria (e.g., aromatic amine-induced papilloma).

(*g*) *Aminoaciduria.* Tubular deficit induced by some metals (e.g., cadmium) may result in aminoaciduria. In the normal adult, urinary excretion of aminoacids does not exceed 200 mg of α-aminonitrogen in 24 hours.

(*h*) *Enzymuria.* Under normal conditions, the enzymes present in urine may originate from three sources:

—serum (enzymes of low molecular mass ($< 400\,000$), such as lysozyme and ribonuclease);
—desquamated epithelial cells of the urogenital tract (these usually appear in insignificant quantities);
—secretions of the urogenital tract glands (these are more important in males than in females).

In kidney damage, cellular enzymes are released into the tubular lumen. Their determination in urine may indicate the extent of kidney damage, particularly in acute toxic tubular necrosis from long-term exposure to agents such as cadmium and mercury vapour.

However, on an individual basis, the usefulness of urinary enzyme determination in the early detection of kidney injury following long-term exposure to nephrotoxic chemicals is rather limited. This is due to factors that modify the activity of the enzymes in urine samples, namely:

—high inter- and intra-individual variability;
—interference of various factors (inhibitors, activators) in the normal activities of enzymes; and
—storage conditions of urine samples (temperature, pH, bacterial growth).

(i) *Cytological examination of urine*. Regular screening of urine samples for the presence of transformed cells may be indicated in workers exposed to urinary tract carcinogens (e.g., some aromatic amines).

(2) *Blood analyses*

Blood urea nitrogen (BUN), creatinine, β_2-microglobulin. In detecting impairment of glomerular filtration rate, the determination of blood urea nitrogen is usually considered to be a less sensitive method than the determination of plasma creatinine. In the absence of malignant diseases, β_2-microglobulin in serum is a very sensitive indicator of impaired glomerular filtration rate. Creatinine measurement is not recommended for screening purposes.

Tests of urinary system function

These tests are performed only when the screening tests suggest the presence of renal dysfunction. They measure glomerular permeability (glomerular filtration rate), renal plasma flow, proximal tubular function (e.g., reabsorption of glucose, bicarbonate and phosphate, 24-hour excretion of calcium), and distal tubular function (e.g., acidification test).

The creatinine-clearance test (urine collected for 2 hours) deserves a special mention. Serial measurements in workers in whom some screening tests are abnormal may provide an indication of the direction of renal function changes. The advantages of the creatinine-clearance test are that it can be performed under good technical control and that a complete urine collection can be successfully obtained over a short period of time.

Other tests

Renal biopsy using light and electron microscopy, immunological studies of the specimens, and radioisotopic and radiographic examination of the kidney are useful in frankly pathological cases.

Application and usefulness

The tests described above do not cause any inconvenience to the workers, and can be performed by most clinical laboratories. For routine screening of workers subject to long-term exposure to nephrotoxic chemicals, only the most relevant tests need to be carried out. The selection of appropriate tests must be based on the types of nephrotoxin to which the workers are exposed. For example, the regular detection of microscopic haematuria is imperative for workers exposed to certain aromatic amines, whereas the regular determination of specific proteins in urine is indicated for workers exposed to nephrotoxic metals.

CHAPTER 35

The cardiovascular system

Function

The essential function of the cardiovascular system is to circulate blood through the entire body.

Pathophysiological mechanisms

In acute poisonings, cardiac damage may occur in two ways: (*a*) by direct action on heart muscle or on the heart conductive system (e.g., the effect of halogenated hydrocarbons on the heart); and (*b*) as a result of tissue hypoxia (carbon monoxide, hydrogen sulfide, hydrogen cyanide).

Although similar types of effect may exist in long-term low-level exposures, the major concern is the enhanced development of atherosclerosis followed by ischaemic changes in vital organs (brain, heart) (see Chapter 16).

The pathophysiology of vibration-induced vascular changes in the hands has not yet been clarified. Both direct harmful effects on the vascular walls and reflex vasospastic mechanisms triggered through nervous receptors are believed to play a role.

Common disorders and differential diagnosis

It must be stressed that many of the cardiovascular manifestations related to occupational exposures are often precipitated by an underlying pathology of non-occupational origin. In individual workers it is extremely difficult, if not impossible, to prove that occupational factors are responsible for cardiovascular disorders. In groups of workers, however, it is sometimes possible to demonstrate a relationship between an increased occurrence of cardiovascular disorders and occupational factors.

Cardiac affections

Coronary heart disease. Excess morbidity and mortality due to ischaemic heart disease has been well established in workers exposed to

236

carbon disulfide in the viscose rayon industry. The multifarious cardiovascular syndrome of chronic carbon disulfide poisoning includes, in addition to ischaemic heart disease, elevated blood pressure, disturbances in the retinal microcirculation, retinal microaneurysms (in some populations), and the impairment of central nervous system function due to both direct toxic and vascular effects. Since carbon disulfide does not cause any pathognomonic cardiovascular symptoms, confirmation of the etiology of cardiovascular disease is usually impossible in individual carbon disulfide workers, and the probability that the findings are occupation-related has to be based on the exposure history and on the diverse manifestations of carbon disulfide poisoning.

The presence in the blood of carboxyhaemoglobin (in exposure to carbon monoxide or methylene chloride, the metabolite of which is carbon monoxide) or of methaemoglobin (in exposure to aromatic amino and nitro derivatives) diminishes the oxygen supply to the tissues. In subjects with pre-existing coronary atherosclerosis, acute signs of myocardial ischaemia (angina pectoris, myocardial infarction) may develop. Similarly, dysfunction of other organs affected by atherosclerosis may appear (e.g., cerebrovascular disorders, intermittent claudication in the legs).

Cardiac arrhythmias. Exposure to fluoroalkanes, notably trichlorofluoromethane (FC 11), may give rise to cardiac arrhythmias. Evidence from animal experiments and clinical case reports points to some link between certain other organic solvents (trichloroethylene, 1,1,1-trichloroethane, benzene, toluene, heptane) and increased myocardial irritability, manifesting as paroxysmal atrial fibrillation, premature atrial contractions, increased frequency of premature ventricular beats, and ventricular fibrillation. The clinical significance of these potentially arrhythmogenic chemicals remains largely unexplored at workplaces. In workers who had suffered from arrhythmia following exposure to certain organic solvents, the resting electrocardiograms were found to be normal.

Sudden death. Sudden death may be defined as natural death that occurs unexpectedly within 6 hours (or within 24 hours depending on the criteria used) of the onset of the terminal event. The most common causes of sudden death are cardiovascular diseases, notably atherosclerotic coronary artery disease. Instantaneous sudden death is thought to be caused almost invariably by arrhythmia.

Exposure to organic nitrates for a few years in the explosives industry has resulted in severe cases of angina and sudden cardiac death shortly (1–2 days) after the cessation of exposure (see Chapter 19).

Chronic cor pulmonale. The chronic form of cor pulmonale (with or without heart failure) is characterized by hypertrophy and dilatation of the right ventricle owing to an increase in pressure in the pulmonary circulation. It may result from the involvement of lung vasculation in the course of fibrotic reaction to dusts, such as silica, asbestos, coal, and organic materials. It may also result from hypoventilation in patients with chronic bronchitis or emphysema with or without other occupational lung disorders (usually late in the course of the disease).

Affections of peripheral blood vessels

Secondary Raynaud's phenomenon. Several years' exposure to vibrating tools (e.g., chain-saws, pneumatic drills, or chisels) may result in vasospastic disease of the hands caused by pathological changes in the peripheral microcirculation. The condition is characterized by temporary whitening, tingling, and numbness of the fingers of the hand, especially in cold weather. The diagnosis is based on an occupational history of vibration exposure and characteristic symptomatology.

Autoclave cleaners in the vinyl chloride polymerization process may develop Raynaud's phenomenon associated with acro-osteolysis of the terminal phalanges of the hands.

Tests

The history of symptoms remains a cornerstone of the diagnosis of cardiovascular disorders. Thoughtful questioning regarding the pattern of the principal symptoms—such as chest pain, dyspnoea, palpitation, syncope, cough, oedema, and fatigue—is usually the best way of collecting information about cardiovascular disorders, especially when it is combined with an adequate physical examination that includes inspection, palpation, and auscultation.

A 12-lead electrocardiogram is frequently informative in the diagnosis of various manifestations of ischaemic heart disease and different types of circulatory disturbance. In suspected ischaemic heart disease, the diagnostic accuracy of the electrocardiogram can be improved by combining the recording with an exercise test or by carrying out a 24-hour (Halter) recording of the electrocardiogram at the workplace.

Ordinary chest radiographs may indicate the presence of certain diseases of the heart and great vessels (e.g., established cor pulmonale), but they are of little value in early detection. The same is true for biochemical alterations, which may occur in the blood in myocardial infarction. Probably the most useful tests for cor pulmonale resulting from fibrosis are the DCO and ventilation tests.

The procedure for the examination of hands in vibration-induced vasospastic disorders is described in Chapter 24.

CHAPTER 36

The locomotor system

Functions

The locomotor system is responsible for the performance of voluntary movements and ensures harmonious coordination between the supportive structures (bones), the joints, tendons, and muscles, and the nervous system.

Pathophysiological mechanisms

Localized vibration of body parts causes a wide variety of disorders, ranging from neurovascular disorders to degenerative changes of muscles and connective tissues. It is probable, that the pathological changes caused by vibrations are non-linear and depend on the energy absorbed by the hands from the tool. Thus, the characteristics of vibration and the way the tool is used affect the eventual outcome.

Pneumatic tools, hand-guided rock drills, and power chain-saws are the most common sources of local vibration. Osteoarticular disorders in decompression disease are mainly due to the formation of nitrogen bubbles in the tissues, leading to obstruction of the blood circulation. There are also other deleterious effects, for instance, on the coagulation of blood, which may contribute to hypoxic infarction of joints.

Some chemicals may directly affect bone metabolism, causing osteoporosis and pseudofractures (cadmium), exostoses, areas of hypo- and hypermineralization (fluorine), and acro-osteolysis (vinyl chloride) in the distal parts of the fingers. Secondary osteoporotic changes may develop as a result of chronic renal insufficiency in occupational affections of the kidneys.

Common disorders and differential diagnosis

Vibration (local) may cause osteoarthritic changes, particularly in the wrist bones, elbow, and acromioclavicular joint. Bone vacuoles, cysts, and decalcification zones also develop frequently. Muscle and tendon affections often appear as epicondylitis or tendosynovitis. Dysbaric osteonecrosis mostly occurs in the large joints (knee, thigh, shoulder).

239

Since some degeneration of muscles, joints, etc. is part of the normal aging process, the attribution of an occupational etiology to musculoskeletal diseases is usually difficult. However, if attention is paid to the following points, the confirmation of the etiology may be facilitated:

—Pain is often the most important sign of musculoskeletal disorders (which as such is not easily quantifiable). In itai-itai disease, which is endemic in Japan, osteoporosis is accompanied by severe pain.
—Occupation-related musculoskeletal disorders usually develop in younger age groups, while non-occupational osteoarthritis and other forms of degeneration of the joints and muscles develop later in life. An exception to this rule is cadmium poisoning, in which osteoporosis, osteomalacia, and pseudofractures, though rare, occur late in life.
—In the case of vibration-related disorders, the condition is usually localized unilaterally to the body parts most exposed to vibration.

Radiological findings are the earliest signs, whereas stiffening of the vertebral column (poker back) is a late manifestation. Bands in the neck of the teeth are sometimes found as signs of excessive cadmium exposure, and marbled teeth sometimes indicate fluorine intoxication. Vinyl-chloride-induced acro-osteolysis in polyvinyl chloride autoclave cleaners is discussed in Chapter 17.

Functional disturbances in the locomotor system do not usually become manifest until the later stages of the disease process. Thus, their detection is of little value in the early diagnosis of occupation-related locomotor disorders.

Tests

Medical history and physical examination (limitation of movements) are the main tools for the detection of musculotendinous affections. Radiography is the only means of diagnosing skeletal disorders but is of value only in rather advanced stages.

Environmental assessment and biological monitoring

CHAPTER 37

Procedures for environmental assessment of exposure

Some knowledge of the procedures used in the assessment of exposure to harmful substances in the workplace is essential in deciding on the need for periodic preventive health examinations and on their scope and frequency. Although such measurements are not usually carried out by health personnel responsible for preventive health examinations, a good understanding of this field is indispensable for all those involved in occupational health.

Objectives of assessment of exposure

There are three main objectives of assessment of exposure:

—to determine the level of exposure of workers to harmful agents;
—to assess the need for control measures; and
—to ensure the efficiency of control measures in use.

The realization of these objectives depends greatly on the methods selected for sampling and analysis, since sometimes there may be shortcomings due to, for example, poor sensitivity of the available analytical methods.

Exposure assessment procedures

The assessment of hazards in the working environment consists of (*a*) determination of the levels of hazardous agents in the workplace; and (*b*) comparison of the results obtained with adopted exposure limits.

The former involves different types of measurement and analysis:

—measurement of levels of hazards such as noise and radiation;
—measurement of environmental factors such as temperature, humidity, and air movements;
—measurement of the concentrations of airborne contaminants (e.g., gases, vapours, and particles);
—collection of air samples for further analysis in a laboratory (e.g., certain types of dust and chemicals).

Regarding the comparison of the measured concentrations with established exposure limits, it should be pointed out that only a very limited number of these exposure limits is based on valid information. The majority of the limits are not definitive and change constantly as and when new information becomes available.

Steps in assessment of exposure

The first step is to identify the hazards by carefully observing work processes, machinery, raw materials used, by-products, potential hazards, work practices, etc.

The next step is to design a strategy of sampling, giving priority to the most significant hazards (in terms of toxicity or ability to cause health impairment, possibility of exposure, and number of workers exposed) and to obtaining representative samples.

In factories where production is continuous there is less change in levels of harmful agents during the work-shifts compared with industries in which the operations are cyclic, sporadic, or irregular or when the production programmes are alternating. In the latter cases, the concentrations and duration of workers' exposure to the harmful agents are liable to continual changes. However, even in apparently constant situations, the concentrations of airborne contaminants can vary because of, for example, changes in ambient conditions and slight variations in the process. These factors must be taken into account in designing measurements and techniques for sampling and analysis and in selecting the location, time, and duration of sampling and the number of measurements or samples.

The above considerations refer to the evaluation of airborne pollutants. For physical agents, similar strategies aiming at the representative evaluation of exposures should be followed, keeping in mind the differences between the two types of evaluation.

The location of sampling will depend on its objective. If workers' exposures are to be determined, the samples should be taken in their breathing zone (defined as the front part of a sphere of 30 cm radius around the worker's head). If the objective is to locate and evaluate pollution sources or determine the efficiency of control measures, general workroom samples should be taken from appropriate locations (area sampling).

Personal sampling is the preferred method for evaluating individual exposure. In this method, a sampling device is worn by the worker. The device usually consists of a pump, which is hooked on to the worker's belt or pocket, and a sampling head containing the collecting device (e.g., sorbent tube or filter), which is clipped on to the worker's clothing. Recently, passive samplers have been developed and are already being widely used in certain countries; these consist of a collection tube that allows diffusion of the toxic gas or vapour, which is adsorbed on to a solid sorbent.

When personal sampling is not feasible, it is still possible to make an approximate measurement of a worker's exposure by collecting an area sample in the breathing zone of the worker. In the case of workers who work at different sites at different times, the sampling unit could be carried to different locations and the sample inlet held in the breathing zone of the worker; in field conditions this is, however, very difficult.

There is usually a mixture of agents present in the working environment. After the individual components have been identified, their relative importance as health hazards, as well as the impact of their combination, have to be evaluated. For the evaluation of exposure to aerosols (i.e., airborne particulate matter) it is necessary to determine also the frequency distribution of particles according to size, particularly the fraction smaller than 5 µm (respirable fraction). In interpreting simultaneous exposure to several agents, the mode of action of the different agents must be taken into account. Although possible interactions of substances are extremely complex, it has been the custom to accept several simplifying assumptions. If the effects of the different hazards can be considered as additive, the sum of the concentrations (C_n) of each substance as a fraction of its exposure limit (T_n) should not exceed 1:

$$\frac{C_1}{T_1} + \frac{C_2}{T_2} + \ldots \frac{C_n}{T_n} \leqslant 1$$

This would be the case in exposure to, for example, a mixture of organic solvents that have narcotic effects.

When the chief effects of the different harmful substances are not additive but independent, exposure is judged by comparing the actual concentrations to each exposure limit.

$$\frac{C_1}{T_1} \leqslant 1, \text{ and } \frac{C_2}{T_2} \leqslant 1, \ldots \frac{C_n}{T_n} \leqslant 1$$

This situation may be encountered in, for example, a mine where dust and carbon monoxide may be present simultaneously. Other interpretations are also possible, but in general it should be recognized that disease from one cause may sometimes lessen resistance to other harmful agents.

The time of sampling will vary depending on the type of work process. The following factors should be taken into account in deciding on the time of sampling: (*a*) the type of production process; (*b*) presence of sporadic operations (e.g., repairs, maintenance); (*c*) variations in physical ambient conditions (e.g., temperature, air movement); (*d*) location and movement of workers; and (*e*) work practices.

In exposure to agents whose effect is chronic and/or cumulative, (e.g., silica dust, lead) long-term (several hours or the whole work-shift) sampling is adequate. When dealing with substances that may cause acute poisoning, sampling should be designed so as to detect peaks in concentrations. Short-term sampling (using direct-reading instruments, whenever possible) is recommended for this purpose. The duration of sampling will also be dictated by the minimum amount of substance required for each analytical method.

The results of repeated measurements vary not only because of fluctuations in the environmental concentrations of pollutants, but also as a result of imperfections in the collection and analysis of samples. The greater the discrepancies between repeated measurements, the larger the number of samples required to make an estimate of the true average concentration.

It should be noted that the accuracy and precision of environmental evaluation should correspond to the objectives of the evaluation. In workplaces where concentrations are expected to be 10 times the adopted exposure limits, it is not necessary to spend resources on extremely accurate and precise methodology in order to establish the need for implementation of control measures. Even if the actual concentration were estimated with some error, the practical conclusion would still be that control measures were needed. However, since nowadays hazardous agents are better controlled and workplaces are improving to a point where concentrations remain low or undectable, very precise instruments, highly sensitive methods, and appropriate statistical procedures are becoming more and more necessary.

Most countries have adopted exposure limits as time-weighted average concentrations (i.e., the average concentration during five 8-hour work-shifts per week). In addition, frequently there are short-term (usually 15-min) exposure limits for acute exposure. A sampling strategy that aims at comparing the actual concentrations with exposure limits must respect the definition of exposure limits.

Considering the mobility of workers and possible unforeseen exposures, including those occurring outside the workplace, it is important, whenever possible, to complement the environmental evaluation of exposures with biological assessment, particularly if the agents are known to enter the body by routes other than inhalation, such as through ingestion or skin absorption.

CHAPTER 38

Biological monitoring of exposure

Objectives

The biological monitoring of exposure has two aims: (*a*) to measure the concentrations of harmful agents and their metabolites in biological samples[1] of exposed individuals; and (*b*) to determine the intensity of biochemical and histological changes due to exposure (e.g., inhibition of acetylcholinesterase by organophosphorus compounds).

The first aim involves the analysis of one or more indicators of exposure in representative biological samples. The second aim is not concerned with the evaluation of exposure but with the detection of early biochemical and physical changes in exposed workers.

Important considerations in biological monitoring

Kinetics of absorption and excretion

The rate of absorption of a harmful agent is influenced by the environmental conditions at the workplace. For example, the total amount of a substance absorbed in the lungs depends on: (*a*) the concentration of the agent in the workroom air, the duration of exposure, and the rates of pulmonary ventilation and retention; and (*b*) the chemical and physical properties of the agent.

The rate at which different toxic substances are excreted determines their biological half-life—i.e., the time during which half of the total amount of an absorbed harmful agent is eliminated from the body (or from the biological samples).

The half-lives of harmful industrial agents may be divided into three categories: short (several hours—e.g., furfural, phenol, toluene, xylene); medium (several tens of hours—e.g., perchloroethylene, trichloroethylene); and long (several weeks or even months—e.g., mercury, lead).

Substances with a short biological half-life (e.g., two hours) are excreted rapidly after the end of exposure. Their concentration in body fluids or tissues or in exhaled air drops practically to zero within

---

[1] Body fluids, tissues, and excretory products.

approximately 16 hours. Substances having a medium biological half-life (e.g., 48 hours) are fully excreted in a relatively longer time (one week or more). When the concentration of a substance is being measured in a person who is exposed to the agent in question daily, it is clear that part of the concentration measured may be the contribution of the previous day's exposure. Moreover, after several days of exposure, a dynamic equilibrium is established, in which the amount of the substance excreted is the same as that absorbed during exposure. The excretion rate oscillates between two extreme values, the maximum and minimum being at the end and beginning of the workshift, respectively. The same applies to substances with a long biological half-life; however, the establishment of equilibrium takes a very long time and the daily oscillations are very slight.

Metabolism

The fate of the harmful agent in the body (i.e., the result of the metabolic changes the agent undergoes in the body) is an important factor in biological assessment. A knowledge of the metabolic pathways of harmful agents is useful in selecting the appropriate medium for biological testing. For example, certain chemicals or their metabolites may be more easily tested in urine than in blood.

Relationship between exposure and concentration of harmful agents in biological samples

The mean concentration of a harmful agent in the inhaled air may serve as a measure of exposure. However, such a measure is far from ideal because it takes no account of individual differences in pulmonary ventilation, which varies greatly at different workloads.

It is preferable to express the level of exposure in terms of the dose of the chemical retained in the body during a workshift. The results are unrelated to lung ventilation and there is usually a good correlation between the amount absorbed and the level of the chemical substance in biological samples. However, this relationship can be studied only under laboratory conditions.

Analytical methods and their sensitivity and selectivity

The methods of biological assessment are frequently complex and include, for example, chromatography, high-pressure liquid chromatography, and atomic absorption spectrophotometry.

Tests based on urine analysis

Urine has the advantage of ease of collection. Exogenous chemicals or their metabolites are often excreted in the urine in amounts proportional to the absorbed dose.

Sampling

The selection of the type of urine sample depends on (*a*) the half-life of the agent to be monitored; (*b*) the conditions of exposure (whether the concentration of the chemical in air was constant or variable); and (*c*) the required accuracy of the exposure test.

Whole-day sample. All the urine excreted during 24 hours from the start of the workshift. Although whole-day samples are desirable for high accuracy in estimating exposure, they are impracticable to collect on a routine basis.

Whole-workshift sample. Urine excreted during the workshift. Such a sample is easily collected under field conditions and is a suitable compromise between the whole-day and short-term sample.

Short-term sample. Urine excreted during the last two hours of the workshift. It is recommended for monitoring compounds with long or medium biological half-lives. For compounds with short biological half-lives, it is suitable only if their air concentration is more or less constant throughout the workshift; otherwise the urine concentration reflects predominantly the air concentration immediately preceding sampling.

End-of-workshift sample. The sample collected at the end of a workshift. This type of sample is recommended for assessing exposure to substances with a long or medium biological half-life. The results of the analysis must be corrected to standard urine density or grams of creatinine.

Morning-after sample. Urine collected in the morning before the start of the workshift. This is usually used in very selected cases (e.g., exposure to fluorine). The results of the analysis must be corrected to standard urine density or grams of creatinine.

Expressing the results of urine analysis

The results of urine analyses can be expressed in several ways:

Concentration in mg/litre or mmol/litre. These are the simplest and most commonly used units. However, the concentrations of chemicals in the urine of individuals exposed to the same air concentrations are largely dependent on the volume of excreted urine, which varies according to the intake and losses of water, and these are in turn influenced by factors such as temperature and physical exertion.

Concentration data converted to standard urine density. The following urine density standards are usually used: 1.016, 1.020, or 1.024 g/ml at 20 °C. (The standards differ because the mean density of urine varies in different population groups.) Results corrected to standard urine density are less variable than the simple, uncorrected concentration data. Correction is particularly recommended for compounds with long or medium biological half-lives and for ill-defined samples (e.g., end-of-workshift).

Concentration data converted to creatinine. This is another method of standardizing concentration data. In this case the amount of hazardous agent or its metabolite(s) (in mg) is corrected to 1 g of creatinine, which is excreted at a relatively steady rate.

Excretion rate. This measurement is expressed in mg/hour. It is valid only when the urine sample is collected over a defined period (whole-day or whole-workshift samples). In order to avoid confusion, it is best to state the amount of the substance and the time period of sampling—e.g., mg/2 hours (during the last two hours of the workshift), mg/8 hours (during the workshift), and mg/24 hours. In many cases of continuous exposure, the excretion rate is a highly accurate measure of the daily exposure level.

Precision of biological assessment of exposure

A well controlled exposure test can, as a rule, give results repeatable to within $\pm 20\%$; few environmental methods of exposure assessment yield better or as good results.

Exposure tests based on blood analysis

Blood analysis is rarely used for the purposes of biological monitoring in industrial situations owing to the difficulty of obtaining frequent samples. It is reserved for those occupational health problems that cannot be solved by urine or breath monitoring. Some of the exceptions are the analysis of lead and zinc protoporphyrin in blood (in lead exposure) and cholinesterase activity in blood (in exposure to organophosphorus compounds).

Exposure tests based on analysis of exhaled air

These tests permit the assessment of the level of exposure to volatile industrial chemicals that are not metabolized (or are metabolized to a small degree only)[1] and that predominantly eliminated from the body in exhaled air. These include, for example, methylchloroform, perchloroethylene and other halogenated hydrocarbons.

Breath analyses are done on samples of either alveolar air (collected towards the end of the workshift) or total exhaled air in one breath. Since in the early post-exposure period the concentration of the inhaled chemical in exhaled air drops sharply, even small differences in sampling time may cause a great difference in the obtained concentration values. It appears, therefore, that sampling in the early post-exposure period should be avoided; rather, it should be done some time after the termination of exposure. The most appropriate

---

[1] These tests are not recommended for rapidly metabolized substances (e.g., toluene, xylene), because only a small amount of the retained dose is eliminated by exhalation and the concentration of the substance in the exhaled air decreases rapidly below the limit of reliable measurement.

time can be reliably determined only on the basis of a good knowledge of the process of respiratory elimination of the substance in question.

Exposure tests based on the analysis of expired air have not attained the precision of exposure tests based on urine analysis, since in the case of breath analysis, the results may be influenced by a number of factors, such as different durations of exposure, mode of sampling, the time of sampling, and physical activity during the interval between the end of exposure and sampling. In spite of these drawbacks, breath analysis remains a useful complementary test to other biological and environmental methods of assessment of exposure to industrial chemicals.

Significance of biological tests

Biological tests are highly sensitive indices of an individual's exposure and they have become an effective and powerful tool for the industrial hygienist. They give information on the overall level of exposure, regardless of whether the industrial chemical has entered the organism by the respiratory, oral, or cutaneous route. Cutaneous absorption can play a significant role in the case of some organic compounds; the amounts absorbed through the skin may be comparable to or even higher than those that enter the body through the respiratory tract. In manufacturing premises, environmental control measures should be supplemented, wherever possible, with biological tests on workers. Knowledge of the real individual exposure permits flexible application of various preventive measures, which are often more effective and less expensive than general reduction of the concentration of toxic substances in the workroom air.

Bibliography

The text of this manual is based on monographs in the field of occupational health published in the last decade, and only exceptional reference is made to older works or to single papers. This bibliography is also intended to serve as a list of publications recommended as further reading.

General references

1. ARTAMONOVA, V. G. ET AL. *Vračebnotrudovaja ekspertiza i reabilitacijapri professional'nyh zabolevanijah* [*Medical assessment of work-ability and rehabilitation in occupational diseases*]. Leningrad, Medicina, 1975 (in Russian).
2. BROWNING, E. *Toxicity and metabolism of industrial solvents*. Amsterdam, Elsevier, 1965.
3. BROWNING, E. *Toxicity of industrial metals*, 2nd ed. London, Butterworth, 1969.
4. CHIAPPINO, G. & TOMASINI, M. *Medicina e igiene del lavoro* [*Occupational medicine and hygiene*]. Milano, Libreria Cortine, 1979 (in Italian).
5. CLAYTON, G. D. & CLAYTON, F. E., ED. *Patty's industrial hygiene and toxicology*. Vol. 2. New York, John Wiley & Sons, 1981.
6. CRALLEY, L. V. ET AL. ED. *Industrial environmental health; the worker and community*. New York, Academic Press, 1972.
7. DESOILLE, H. ET AL. ED. *Précis de médecine du travail* [*Review of occupational medicine*]. Paris, Masson, 1980 (in French).
8. GARDNER, G. W., ED. *Current approaches to occupational health. 2*. Bristol, Wright, 1982.
9. GRACIANSKAJA, L. A. ET AL. *Socialno-trudovaja i medicinskaja reabilitacija bol'nych professional'nymi zabolevanijami* [*Social work and medical rehabilitation of patients with occupational diseases*]. Leningrad, Medicina, 1978 (in Russian).
10. GRACIANSKAJA, L. N. & KOVŠILO, V. E. ED. *Spravočnik po professionalnoj patologii.* [*Handbook on occupational pathology*]. Leningrad, Medicina, 1981 (in Russian).
11. GRANDJEAN, P. *Occupational health aspects of construction work*. Copenhagen, WHO Regional Office for Europe, 1983 (EURO Reports and Studies, No. 86).
12. HAGUENOER, J. M. ET AL. *Les cancers professionnels* [*Occupational cancers*]. Paris, Technique et Documentation—Lavoisier, 1982.
13. HENSCHLER, H., ED. *Gesundheitsschädliche Arbeitsstoffe* [*Harmful substances in the workplace*]. Weinheim, Verlag Chemie, 1981 (in German).

14. *IARC Monographs on the evaluation of the carcinogenic risk of chemicals to humans; chemicals, industrial processes and industries associated with cancer in humans.* Lyon, International Agency for Research on Cancer, 1982 (IARC Monographs Supplement 4 and IARC Monographs, Vol. 1–29).
15. INTERNATIONAL LABOUR ORGANISATION. *Occupational exposure limits for airborne toxic substances.* Second (revised) edition. Geneva, International Labour Office, 1980. (Occupational Safety and Health Series, No. 37).
16. IZMEROV, N. F., ED. *Rukovodstvo po professionalnym zabolevanijam.* [*Handbook of occupational diseases*]. Moscow, Medicina, 1983 (in Russian).
17. KEY, M. M. ET AL. ED. *Occupational diseases: a guide to their recognition.* Washington, DC, Department of Health, Education and Welfare, 1977 (NIOSH Publication, No. 77–181).
18. KOELSCH, F., ED. *Handbuch der Berufskrankheiten* [*Handbook of occupational diseases*]. Jena, Fischer, 1972 (in German).
19. KUNDIEV, JU. I. & KRASNJUK, E. P., ED. *Professional'nye zabolevanija rabotnikov sel'skogo hozajstva* [*Occupational diseases in agricultural workers*]. Kiev, Zdorov'ja, 1983 (in Russian).
20. LAUWERYS, R. *Toxicologie industrielle et intoxications professionnelles* [*Industrial toxicology and occupational intoxications*]. 2nd ed. Paris, Masson, 1982 (in French).
21. LAZAREV, N. V., ED. *Vrednye veščestva v promyšlennosti* [*Hazardous substances in industry*]. Leningrad, Chimia, 1977 (in Russian).
22. McDONALD, J. C., ED. Recent advances in occupational health. Edinburgh, Churchill—Livingstone, 1981.
23. MAKOTČENKO, V. M. ET AL. ED. *Gigiena truda i profilaktika profzabolevanij v metalloobrabatyvajuščej promyšlennosti* [*Industrial hygiene and prevention of occupational diseases in the metal-processing industry*]. Kiev, Zdorov'ja, 1979 (in Russian).
24. MEDVED, L. I. & KUNDIEV, JU. I., ED. *Gigiena truda v selskohozajstvennom proizvodstve* [*Industrial hygiene in agricultural production*]. Moscow, Medicina, 1981 (in Russian).
25. PIDPALYI, G. P. ET AL. ED. *Professional'nye zabolevanija rabočich gornorudnoj promyšlennosti* [*Occupational diseases in mining-industry workers*]. Kiev, Zdorov'ja, 1981 (in Russian).
26. RAŠEVSKAJA, A. M. ET AL. *Professional'nye bolezni* [*Occupational diseases*]. Moscow, Medicina, 1973 (in Russian).
27. ROM, W. N. ED. *Environmental and occupational medicine.* Boston, Little Brown and Company, 1983.
28. SCHILLING, R. S. F., ED. *Occupational health practice.* 2nd edition. London, Butterworth, 1981.
29. SEREBROV, A. I. & DANECKAJA, O. L. *Professional'nye novoobrazovanija* [*Occupational tumours*]. Leningrad, Medicina, 1976 (in Russian).
30. *Women and occupational health risks. Report on a WHO meeting.* Copenhagen WHO Regional Office for Europe, 1983 (EURO Reports and Studies, No. 76).
31. ZENZ, C., ED. *Occupational medicine.* Chicago, Year Book Medical Publishers, 1975.

Respiratory system and its disorders

1. Commission of European Communities; Working Group of Experts. *Public health risks of exposure to asbestos.* Oxford, Pergamon Press, 1977.

2. DUBININA, V. P. *Silikotuberkulez* [*Silicotuberculosis*]. Moscow, Medicina, 1978 (in Russian).
3. FISH, J. E. Occupational asthma: a spectrum of acute respiratory diseases. *Journal of occupational medicine*, **24**: 379–386 (1982).
4. GERNEZ-RIEUX, C. ET AL. *Broncho-pneumopathies professionnelles* [*Occupational bronchopulmonary diseases*]. Paris, Masson, 1961 (in French).
5. HEALTH AND SAFETY EXECUTIVE. *Report of Advisory Committee on Asbestos*. London, H.M. Stationery Office, 1979.
6. HENDRICK, D. J. & WEILL, H. Acute reactions to inhaled agents. In: McDonald, J. C., ed. *Recent advances in occupational health*. Edinburgh, Churchill—Livingstone, 1981, pp. 39–50.
7. *Asbestos*. Lyon, International Agency for Research on Cancer, 1976 (IARC Monographs on the Evaluation of Carcinogenic Risk of Chemicals to Man, Vol. 14.)
8. INTERNATIONAL LABOUR ORGANISATION. *Guidelines for the use of ILO international classification of radiographs of the pneumoconioses*. Geneva, International Labour Office, 1980 (Occupational Safety and Health Series, No. 22 (Rev. 80)).
9. KARAPATA, A. P. & ŠEVČENKO, A. M. *Professional'nye pylevye bolezni legkih* [*Occupational dust diseases of the lung*]. Kiev, Zdorov'ja, 1980 (in Russian).
10. MORGAN, W. K. C. & SEATON, A. *Occupational lung diseases*. Philadelphia, Saunders, 1975.
11. PARKES, W. R. *Occupational lung disorders*. 2nd edition. London, Butterworth, 1982.
12. PEPYS, J. Occupational asthma: an overview. *Journal of occupational medicine*, **24**: 534–538 (1982).
13. TOLOT, F. ET AL. *Les manifestations pulmonaires des métaux durs*. [*Pulmonary affections caused by hard metals*]. *Archives des maladies professionnelles*, **31**: 453–470 (1970) (in French).
14. ULMER, W. T. & REICHEL, J. A., ED. *Pneumokoniosen* [*Pneumoconioses*]. Berlin, Springer, 1976 (in German).
15. ULMER, W. T. ET AL. *Die Lungenfunktion; Physiologie und Pathophysiologie; Methodik.* [*Lung functions; physiology and pathophysiology; methods*]. Stuttgard, Thieme, 1976 (in German).
16. WAGNER, J. C. ED. *Biological effects of mineral fibres*. Lyon, International Agency for Research on Cancer, 1980. (Proceedings of a Symposium organized by IARC, the French National Institute of Health and Medical Research and the Medical Research Council Pneumoconiosis Unit, Penarth, UK, held at the International Agency for Research on Cancer, Lyon, France 25–27 September 1979) (IARC Scientific Publication, No. 30).
17. WHO Technical Report Series, No. 684. Geneva, 1983 (*Recommended health-based occupational exposure limits for selected vegetable dusts*: report of WHO Study Group).
18. ZAJABREV, JU. P. ET AL. ED. *Ventilacionnaja funkcija legkih (fiziologija, patofiziologija, metody issledovanija)* [*Ventilation function of lungs (physiology, pathophysiology, investigation methods)*]. Alma-Ata, Nauka, 1980 (in Russian).

Beryllium

1. BURNAZJAN, A. J. ED. *Berillij: toksikologija, gigiena, profilaktika i lecenie berillievyh poraženij* [*Beryllium: toxicology, hygiene, prevention and treatment of beryllium injuries*]. Moscow, Atomizdat, 1980 (in Russian).

2. *IARC Monographs on the evaluation of the carcinogenic risk of chemicals to humans. Chemicals and industrial processes associated with cancer in humans.* Lyon, International Agency for Research on Cancer, 1979 (IARC Monographs Supplement 1.).
3. MOLOKANOV, K. P. ET AL. Berillioz [*Berylliosis*]. Moscow, Medicina, 1972 (in Russian).
4. TEPPER, L. B. ET AL. *Toxicity of beryllium compounds.* New York, Elsevier, 1961.

Cadmium

1. LAUWERYS, R. R., Rapporteur. *CEC criteria (dose/effect relationships) for cadmium.* London, Pergamon Press, 1978.
2. LAUWERYS, R. R. *Health maintenance of workers exposed to cadmium. A guide for physicians.* New York, Cadmium Council, 1979.
3. WHO Technical Report Series, No. 647. Geneva, 1980 (*Recommended health-based limits in occupational exposure to heavy metals*: report of a WHO Study Group).

Phosphorus and its inorganic compounds

1. BERDYHODŽIN, M. T. ET AL. *Ocenka zdorovja rabočih na zavodah pereraboty fosfora.* [*Evaluation of health of workers in phosphorus processing plants*]. *Zdravoohranenie Kazahstana* No. 7: 42–44 (1974) (in Russian).

Organophosphorus compounds

1. BUSLOVIČ, S. JU. & ZAHAROV, G. G. *Klinika i lečenie ostryh otravlenij jadohimikatami (pesticidami)* [*Clinic and therapy of acute poisonings by toxic pesticides*]. Belarus, Minsk, 1972 (in Russian).
2. KAGAN, JU. S. *Toksikologija fosfororganičeskich pesticidov* [*Toxicology of organophosphorus pesticides*]. Medicina, Moscow, 1977 (in Russian).
3. KALOJANOVA-SIMEONOVA, F. *Pesticidy: Toksičeskoe dejstvie i profilaktika* [*Pesticides: toxic effects and prevention*]. Medicina, Moscow, 1980 (in Russian).
4. MEDVED, L. I. ED. *Spravočnik po pesticidam* [*Handbook on pesticides*]. Kiev, Uroszai, 1977 (in Russian).
5. WHO Technical Report Series No. 677. Geneva, 1982 (*Recommended health-based limits in occupational exposure to pesticides*: report of a WHO Study Group).

Chromium

1. HAYES, R. B. Cancer and occupational exposure to chromium chemicals. In: Lilienfeld, A. M. ed. *Reviews in cancer epidemiology*, Vol. 1. New York, Elsevier/North Holland Biomedical Press, 1980.
2. LANGARD, S. & NORSETH, I. Chromium. In: FRIBERG, L. et al. ed. *Handbook of the toxicology of metals.* Amsterdam, Elsevier/North Holland Biomedical Press, 1979.

3. LANGARD, S. Chromium. In: Waldron, H. A. ed. *Metals in the environment.* London, Academic Press, 1980.
4. LANGARD, S. ED. *Biological and environmental aspects of chromium.* Amsterdam, Elsevier/North Holland Biomedical Press, 1982.
5. NATIONAL INSTITUTE FOR OCCUPATIONAL SAFETY AND HEALTH. *Criteria for a recommended standard. Occupational exposure to chromium (VI).* Washington, DC, US Government Printing Office, 1975 (HEW (NIOSH) Publication No. 76–129).

Manganese

1. *Manganese.* Washington, DC, National Academy of Science, 1973.
2. PISCATOR, M. Manganese. In: Friberg, L. ed. *Handbook on the toxicology of metals.* Amsterdam, Elsevier/North Holland Biomedical Press, 1979.
3. ŠARIĆ, M. & LUČIĆ-PALAIĆ, S. Possible synergism of exposure to airborne manganese and smoking habit in occurrence of respiratory symptoms. In: Walton, W. H., ed. Inhaled particles, IV. New York, Pergamon Press, 1977.
4. WHO Technical Report Series No. 647. Geneva, 1980 (*Recommended health-based limits in occupational exposure to heavy metals*: report of a WHO Study Group).
5. *Manganese.* Geneva, World Health Organization, 1981 (Environmental Health Criteria, 17).

Arsenic

1. PINTO, S. S. Arsine poisoning: evaluation of the acute phase. *Journal of occupational medicine,* **18**: 633–635 (1976).
2. *Arsenic.* Geneva, World Health Organization, 1981 (Environmental Health Criteria, 18).

Mercury

1. CLARKSON, T. W. The pharmacology of mercury compounds. *Annual review of pharmacology,* **12**: 375–406 (1972).
2. GOMBOS, B. ET AL. Klinické prejavy u pracovníkov pri výrobe ortuti [*Clinical manifestations in workers in mercury production*]. *Pracovoni Lékarstri,* **27**: 298–301 (1975) (in Slovak).
3. *Mercury.* Geneva, World Health Organization, 1976 (Environmental Health Criteria, 1).
4. WHO Technical Report Series, No. 647. Geneva, 1980 (*Recommended health-based limits in occupational exposure to heavy metals*: report of a WHO Study Group).

Lead

1. BERITIC, T. *Lead and peripheral neuropathy.* Research Triangle Park, Environmental Protection Agency, Office of Research and Development, Health Effects Research Laboratory, 1981.

2. *Lead*. Geneva, World Health Organization, 1977 (Environmental Health Criteria, No. 3).
3. WHO Technical Report Series, No. 647. Geneva, 1980 (*Recommended health-based limits in occupational exposure to heavy metals*: report of a WHO Study Group).

Fluorine

1. *Fluorides: biologic effects of atmospheric pollutants*. Washington, DC, National Academy of Sciences, 1971.
2. SMITH, F. A. & HODGE, H. C. Airborne fluorides and man. In: Strand, K. P. ed. *Critical reviews of environmental control*, Vol. 8. Issue 4 (Part 1). Cleveland, OH, Chemical Rubber Company Press, 1978.
3. *Fluorides and human health*. Geneva, World Health Organization, 1970, (WHO Monograph Series, No. 59).

Carbon disulfide

1. *Carbon disulfide*. Geneva, World Health Organization, 1979 (Environmental Health Criteria, No. 10).
2. WHO Technical Report Series, No. 664, 1981 (*Recommended health-based limits in occupational exposure to selected organic solvents*: report of a WHO Study Group).

Halogenated hydrocarbons

1. BUCKUP, H. *Handlexikon der Arbeitsmedizin [Handbook of occupational medicine]*. Stuttgart, Thieme, 1966 (in German).

Carbon tetrachloride

1. NATIONAL INSTITUTE FOR OCCUPATIONAL SAFETY AND HEALTH. *Criteria for a recommended standard. Occupational exposure to carbon tetrachloride*. Washington, DC, US Government Printing Office, 1975.

Trichloroethylene

1. WHO Technical Report Series, No. 664, 1981 (*Recommended health-based limits in occupational exposure to selected organic solvents*: report of a WHO Study Group).
2. *Trichloroethylene*. Geneva, World Health Organization, 1985 (Environmental Health Criteria, 50).

Polychlorinated biphenyls

1. NATIONAL INSTITUTE FOR OCCUPATIONAL SAFETY AND HEALTH. *Criteria for a recommended standard: occupational exposure to polychlorinated*

biphenyls (PCBs). Washington, DC, US Government Printing Office, 1977.

2. *Polychlorinated biphenyls*. Lyon, International Agency for Research on Cancer, 1978 (IARC Monographs on the Evaluation of the Carcinogenic Risk of Chemicals to Humans, Volume 18).

3. *Polychlorinated biphenyls and terphenyls*. Geneva, World Health Organization, 1976 (Environmental Health Criteria, 2).

Benzene

1. International Workshop on Toxicology of Benzene, Paris, 9th–11th November 1976. *International archives of occupational and environmental health*, **41**: 65–76 (1978).

2. LASKIN, S. & GOLDSTEIN, B. D. ED. Benzene toxicity: a critical evaluation. *Journal of toxicological and environmental health*, Suppl. 2 (1977).

3. *Some industrial chemicals and dyestuffs*. Lyon, International Agency for Research on Cancer, 1982 (IARC Monographs on the Evaluation of the Carcinogenic Risk of Chemicals to Humans, Volume 29).

Toluene

1. WHO Technical Report Series, No. 664, 1981 (*Recommended health-based exposure limits in occupational exposure to selected organic solvents*: report of a WHO Study Group).

2. *Toluene*. Geneva, World Health Organization, 1985 (Environmental Health Criteria, 52).

Xylene

1. WHO Technical Report Series, No. 664, 1981 (*Recommended health-based exposure limits in occupational exposure to selected organic solvents*: report of a WHO Study Group).

Nitroglycerin and nitroglycols

1. NATIONAL INSTITUTE FOR OCCUPATIONAL SAFETY AND HEALTH. *Occupational exposure to nitroglycerine and ethylene glycol dinitrate*. Washington, DC, Department of Health, Education and Welfare, 1978.

Alcohols and ketones

1. *Some fumigants, the herbicides, 2,4-D and 2,4,5-T chlorinated dibenzodioxins and miscellaneous industrial chemicals*. Lyon, International Agency for Research on Cancer, 1977 (IARC Monographs on the Evaluation of the Carcinogenic Risk of Chemicals to Man. Vol. 15).

2. *Selected petroleum products*. Geneva, World Health Organization, 1982 (Environmental Health Criteria, 20).

Carbon monoxide

1. TIUNOV, L. A. & KUSTOV, V. V. *Toksikologija okisi ugleroda* [Toxicology of carbon monoxide]. Moscow, Medicina, 1980 (in Russian).
2. *Selected methods of measuring air pollutants.* Geneva, World Health Organization, 1976 (WHO Offset Publication, No. 24).
3. *Carbon monoxide.* Geneva, World Health Organization, 1979 (Environmental Health Criteria, 13).

Hydrogen cyanide

1. NATIONAL INSTITUTE FOR OCCUPATIONAL SAFETY AND HEALTH. *Criteria for a recommended standard. Occupational exposure to hydrogen cyanide and cyanide salts.* Washington, DC, Department of Health, Education and Welfare, 1976.
2. NATIONAL INSTITUTE FOR OCCUPATIONAL SAFETY AND HEALTH. *Criteria for a recommended standard. Occupational exposure to hydrogen sulfide.* Washington, DC, Department of Health Education and Welfare, 1977.
3. *Hydrogen sulfide.* Geneva, World Health Organization, 1981 (Environmental Health Criteria, No. 19).

Noise

1. NATIONAL INSTITUTE FOR OCCUPATIONAL SAFETY AND HEALTH. *Criteria for a recommended standard. Occupational exposure to noise.* Washington, DC, Department of Health, Education and Welfare, 1973.
2. *Noise.* Geneva, World Health Organization, 1980 (Environmental Health Criteria, 12).

Vibration

1. International Organization for Standardization. *Principles for the measurement and the evaluation of human exposure to vibration transmitted to the hand.* Geneva, ISO, 1976 (ISO/DIS 5349).
2. TAYLOR, W. ED. *The vibration syndrome.* London, Academic Press, 1974.
3. MOLOKANOV, K. P. & SOKOLIK, L. I. *Vlijanie proizvodstvennoj vibracii na kostno—sustavnuju sistemu* [*Influence of industrial vibration on the osteoarticular system*]. Moscow, Medicina, 1978 (in Russian).

Compressed air

1. BENETT, P. B. & ELLIOTT, D. H. *The physiology and medicine of diving and compressed air work.* London, Bailliere Tindall, 1975.

Ionizing radiation

1. *Basic safety standards for radiation protection.* Vienna, International Atomic Energy Agency, 1982 (Report of an advisory group jointly sponsored by IAEA/WHO/ILO/NEA).

2. BRAESTRUP, C. B. & VILKERLÖF, K. J. *Manual on radiation protection in hospitals and general practice.* Vol. 1. *Basic protection requirements.* Geneva, World Health Organization, 1974.
3. *Code of practice on radiation protection of workers in mining and milling of radioactive ores.* Vienna, International Atomic Energy Agency, 1981.
4. GUS'KOVA, A. K. & BAJSOGOLOV, G. D. *Lučevaja bolezň čeloveka* [*Human radiation sickness*]. Moscow, Medicina, 1971 (in Russian).

Skin diseases

1. BRUJEVIČ, T. S. *Professional'nye allergičeskie dermatozy* [*Occupational allergic dermatitis*]. Moscow, Medicina, 1982 (in Russian).
2. CRONIN, E. *Contact dermatitis.* Edinburgh, Churchill-Livingstone, 1980.
3. MAIBACH, H. I. & GELLIN, G. A. *Occupational and industrial dermatology.* London, Year Book Medical Publishers, 1982.

Skin cancer

1. ADAMS, R. M. *Occupational skin disease.* New York, Grune & Stratton, 1983 (Chapter 5).
2. EMMET, E. A. Occupational skin cancer: a review. *Journal of occupational medicine,* **17**: 44–49 (1975).
3. *Selected petroleum products.* Geneva, World Health Organization, 1982 (Environmental Health Criteria, 20).

Infectious and parasitic diseases

1. BENENSON, A. S. ED. *Control of communicable diseases in Man.* Washington, DC, American Public Health Association, 1975.
2. *Code of practice for the prevention of infection in clinical laboratories and post mortem rooms.* London, H.M. Stationery Office, 1978.
3. CONSTABLE, P. J. & HARRINGTON, J. M. The risks of zoonoses in a veterinary service. *British medical journal,* **284**: 246 (23 January 1982).
4. HARRINGTON, J. M. Health and safety in medical laboratories. *Bulletin of the World Health Organization,* **60**: 9–16 (1982).
5. Guidelines for the management of accidents involving microorganisms. A WHO Memorandum. *Bulletin of the World Health Organization,* **58**: 245–256 (1980).
6. NATIONAL INSTITUTE FOR OCCUPATIONAL SAFETY AND HEALTH. *Occupational diseases: a guide to their recognition.* Washington, DC, Department of Health, Education and Welfare, 1977.
7. *Occupational hazards in hospitals. Report on a WHO meeting.* Copenhagen, WHO Regional office for Europe, 1983 (EURO Reports and Studies, No. 80).

Nervous system

1. *Adverse effects of environmental chemicals and psychotropic drugs.* Vol. 2. *Neurophysiological and behavioural tests.* Amsterdam, Elsevier, 1976.

2. CASSITTO, M. G. & FOA, V. Assessment of behavioral toxicology in occupational health. In: Cuomo, & Raccagni, ed. *Applications of behavioral pharmacology in toxicology*. New York, Raven Press (in press).
3. FELDMAN, R. G. ET AL. Neurophysiological effects of industrial toxins: a review. *American journal of industrial medicine*, 1: 211–227 (1980).
4. WHO Technical Report Series No. 654, 1980 (*Peripheral neuropathies*: report of a WHO Study Group).
5. SPENCER, P. S. & SCHAUMBURG, H. H., ED. *Experimental and clinical neurotoxicology*. Baltimore, Williams & Wilkins, 1980.
6. XINTARAS C. ET AL. ED. *Behavioral toxicology: early detection of occupational hazards*. Washington, DC, US Department of Health, Education and Welfare, 1974 (DHEW Publication No. (NIOSH) 74–126).

Blood and blood-forming systems

1. *Manual on radiation haematology*. Technical report series, No. 123. Vienna, International Atomic Energy Agency, 1974.
2. RAŠEVSKAJA, A. M. & ZORINA, L. A. *Professionalnye zabolevanija sistemy krovi* [*Occupational diseases of the blood system*]. Moscow, Medicina, 1968 (in Russian).
3. SOKOLOV, V. V. & GRIBOVA, I. A. *Gematologičeskie pokazateli zdorovogo čeloveka* [*Haematological indices of healthy man*]. Moscow, Medicina, 1972 (in Russian).
4. STOCKINGER, H. E. & MOUNTAIN, J. T. Test for hypersensitivity to haemolytic chemicals. *Archives of environmental health*, 6: 495–502 (1963).
5. *Manual of basic techniques for a health laboratory*. Geneva, World Health Organization, 1980.

Digestive system

1. CREECH, J. L. & JOHNSON, M. H. Angiosarcoma of the liver in the manufacture of polyvinyl chloride. *Journal of occupational medicine*, 16: 150–151 (1974).
2. DAVIDSON, CH. S. ET AL. ED. *Guidelines for detection of hepatotoxicity due to drugs and chemicals*. (NIH Publication No. 79–313). Washington, DC, Department of Health, Education and Welfare, 1979.
3. *Epidemiology studies: screening for the early detection of disease in individuals exposed to vinyl chloride*. Washington, DC, U.S. Environmental Protection Agency, 1981 (Final report No. EPA 560/6–81–002).
4. PLUNKETT, E. R. *Occupational diseases: a syllabus of signs and symptoms*. Stamford, CT, Barret Book Co., 1977.
5. REYNOLDS, E. S. Environmental aspects of injury and disease: liver and bile ducts. *Environmental health perspectives*, 20: 1–13 (1977).

Urinary system

1. LAUWERYS, R. & BERNARD, A. Diagnosis of metal induced nephropathy in humans. *Journal of applied toxicology* (in press).
2. WALKER, H. K. ET AL. *Clinical methods. The history, physical and laboratory examinations*. 2nd ed. London, Butterworth, 1980.

Cardiovascular system

1. BALAZS, T. ED. *Cardiac toxicology.* Boca Raton, FL, CRC Press, 1981.
2. BRAUNWALD, E. ED. *Heart disease. A textbook of cardiovascular medicine.* Philadelphia, Saunders, 1980.
3. KONČALOVSKAJA, N. M. ED. *Serdečno-sosudistaja sistema pri dejstvii promyšlennyh faktorov* [*Cardiovascular system and industrial factors*]. Moscow, Medicina, 1976 (in Russian).
4. TAYLOR, W. & PELNAR, P. L. ED. *Vibration white finger in industry.* London, Academic Press, 1975.

Assessment of exposure

1. BARETTA, E. D. ET AL. Monitoring exposures to vinyl chloride vapour: breath analysis and continuous air sampling. *American Industrial Hygiene Association Journal,* 30: 537 (1969).
2. BASELT, R. C. *Biological monitoring methods for industrial chemicals.* Davis, CA, Biomedical Publications, 1980.
3. BERLIN, A. ET AL. ED. *The use of biological specimens for the assessment of human exposure to environment pollutants.* The Hague, Martinus Nyhoff, 1979.
4. CLAYTON, G. D. & CLAYTON, F. E., ED. *Patty's industrial hygiene and toxicology.* Vol. 1. *General principles.* New York, J. Wiley and Sons, 1978.
5. CRALEY, Z. J. & CRALEY, L. V. ED. *Patty's industrial hygiene and toxicology.* Vol. 3. *Theory and rationale of industrial hygiene practice.* New York, J. Wiley & Sons, 1979.
6. DUTKIEWICZ, T. *Chemia toksykologiczna* [*Toxicological chemistry*]. Warszawa, Pańctwowv Zaklad Wydawnictw Lekarzskich (PZWL) 1974 (in Polish).
7. FERNANDEZ, J. Experimental human exposures to tetrachloroethylene vapor and elimination in breath after inhalation. *American Industrial Hygiene Association Journal,* 37: 143–50 (1976).
8. GADASKINA, I. D. & FILOV, V. A. *Prevraščenie i opredelenie promyšlennyh jadov v organizme* [*The biotransformation and determination of industrial poisons in the body*]. Leningrad, Medicina, 1971 (in Russian).
9. GADASKINA, I. D. ET AL. *Opredelenie neorganičeskih promyšlennyh jadov v organizme.* [*Determination of industrial inorganic poisons in the organism*]. Leningrad, Medicina, 1975 (in Russian).
10. GOLUBEV, A. A. ET AL. *Količestvennaja toksikologija* [*Quantitative toxicology*]. Leningrad, Medicina, 1973 (in Russian).
11. LAUWERYS, R. Biological criteria for selected industrial toxic chemicals: a review. *Scandinavian journal of work, environment and health,* 1: 139–72 (1975).
12. LINCH, A. L. *Biological monitoring for industrial chemical exposure control.* Cleveland, CRC OH, Press, 1974.
13. PIOTROWSKI, J. K. *Exposure tests for organic compounds in industrial toxicology.* Cincinnati, National Institute for Occupational Safety and Health, 1977.
14. SHERWOOD, R. J. & CARTER, F. W. G. The measurement of occupational exposure to benzene vapour. *Annals of occupational hygiene,* 13: 125–46 (1970).
15. STEWART, R. D. ET AL. Experimental human exposure to tetrachloroethylene. *Archives of environmental health,* 20: 224 (1970).

16. STEWART, R. D. ET AL. Human exposure to 1,1,1-trichloroethane vapour: relationship of expired air and blood concentrations to exposure and toxicity. *American Industrial Hygiene Association Journal*, **22**: 252 (1961).
17. TEISINGER, J., ED. *Exposiční testy v průmyslové toxikologii [Exposure tests in industrial toxicology]*. Prague, Avicenum, 1980 (in Czech.).
18. *Evaluation of exposure to airborne particles in the work environment*. Geneva, World Health Organization, 1984 (WHO Offset Publication No. 80).

Annex 1

Questionnaire on respiratory symptoms[1]

General

This questionnaire on respiratory symptoms is a modified version of that approved by the Medical Research Council Committee on Research into Chronic Bronchitis. The object of this questionnaire is to provide information, with as little bias as possible, on the respiratory problems of workers exposed to dusts. The actual wording of each question is given and should be strictly followed. It is easy to see that one might get a different answer to a question phrased "Do you smoke?" than to one phrased "You don't smoke, do you?". In fact even the intonation of the voice may influence a person in his answers. Therefore, one should try to ask the questions in as matter-of-fact way as possible.

The questions should be put fairly quickly so that the replies are those which immediately come to the subject's mind. As far as possible, the subject should answer the questions by saying "yes" or "no", and should be discouraged from trying to amplify or qualify his answers. However, if there is any doubt with regard to any question, the interviewer may briefly discuss that question with the subject. When doubt still remains as to whether the answer should be "yes" or "no", record the answer as "no".

Although the questionnaire may look formidable at first sight, it seldom takes more than 4 minutes to complete.

Comments on individual questions

1. In questions 1, 2, 4, and 5 the word "usually" implies five or more days each week. In questions 3 and 6, "3 months" refers to consecutive months in the winter. When night-shift workers are being interviewed, the words "on getting up" should be used instead of "first thing in the morning" in questions 1 and 4.

2. In calculating the average number of cigarettes smoked per day or grams of tobacco or number of cigars smoked per week (questions

---

[1] Adapted from: BRITISH OCCUPATIONAL HYGIENE SOCIETY COMMITTEE ON HYGIENE STANDARDS (Sub-committee on Vegetable Textile Dusts). A basis for hygiene standards for flax dusts. *Ann. occup. Hyg.*, **23**: 1–26 (1980). For further information on the use of this questionnaire write to: British Medical Research Council, 20 Park Crescent, London W1N 4AL, England.

264

15 and 16), it should be borne in mind that, as a rule, people smoke more at the weekends than on working days.

3. The checklist on occupation is useful to jog the respondent's memory about short periods of work in an industry which might be relevant.

4. In questions 10(a) and 11(a), the word "most" implies on more than 50% of occasions, and the words "first days" refer to every first day back at work after a weekend or holiday.

Questionnaire on respiratory symptoms

		Day	*Month*	*Year*
Work place:				

Name: ....   Date of interview: ....
               (Surname)

               ....   Date of birth: ....
               (First names)

Address: ....   Age: ....   Sex: ....

               ....   Civil state: ....

                                              Race: ....

Social security No ....   Standing height: ....

                                              Weight: ....

                                              Interviewer: ....

Use the actual wording of each question, and record the answers in the boxes provided
(1 = yes; 2 = no; or similar code). When in doubt, record the answer as "no".

Preamble

I am going to ask you some questions, mainly about your chest. I should like you to answer
"yes" or "no" whenever possible.

Cough

(1)   Do you usually cough first thing in the morning?   □

(2)   Do you usually cough during the day or at night?   □

        If "yes" to (1) or (2), ask:

(3a)   Do you cough like this on most days, for as much as 3 months each year?   □

(3b)   Do you cough most on any particular day of the week?   □

(3c)   If "yes", which day(s)?   ....

                                       ....

Phlegm

(4) Do you usually bring up any phlegm from your chest first thing in the morning? □

(5) Do you usually bring up any phlegm from your chest during the day or at night? □

If "yes" to (4) or (5), ask:

(6a) Do you bring up phlegm like this on most days for as much as 3 months each year? □

If "yes" to (6a), ask:

(6b) How long have you had this phlegm? .... years

Periods of cough and phlegm

(7a) In the past 3 years have you had a period of (increased) cough and phlegm lasting for 3 weeks or more? □

If "yes", ask:

(7b) Have you had more than one such period? □

Tightness in chest

(8) Does your chest ever feel tight or your breathing become difficult? □

(9) Do you get this apart from colds? □

If "yes", when? ....

(10) Is your chest tight or your breathing difficult on any particular days? □

If "yes", specify:

    (a) Most of the first days back at work only? □

    (b) Other day(s) also? □

    (c) Only other days? □

If "no" to 10, ask 11:

(11) Has your chest ever been tight or your breathing difficult on any particular days? □

If "yes", specify:

    (a) Most first days back at work only? □

    (b) Other day(s) also? □

    (c) Only other days? □

Breathlessness

If the subject is unable to walk because of any condition other than heart or lung disease, omit question 12 and enter 1 in the box.

(12a) Are you troubled by shortness of breath when hurrying on level ground or walking up a slight hill? □

If "yes", ask:

(12b)   Do you get short of breath walking with other people of your own age on level
         ground?   ☐

         If "yes", ask:

(12c)   Do you have to stop for breath when walking at your own pace on level
         ground?   ☐

(12d)   Is your breathlessness worse on any particular day?   ☐

         If "yes", specify ....

Chest illnesses

(13a)   During the past 3 years have you had any chest illness which has kept you
         away from your usual activities for as much as one week?   ☐

         If "yes", ask:

(13b)   Did you bring up more phlegm than usual during any of these illnesses?   ☐

         If "yes", ask:

(13c)   Have you had more than one illness like this in the past 3 years?   ☐

Past illnesses

Have you ever had:

(14a)   An injury or operation affecting your chest?   ☐

(14b)   Heart trouble?   ☐

(14c)   Bronchitis?   ☐

(14d)   Pneumonia?   ☐

(14e)   Pleurisy?   ☐

(14f)   Pulmonary tuberculosis?   ☐

(14g)   Bronchial asthma?   ☐

(14h)   Other chest trouble?   ☐

(14i)   Hay fever?   ☐

Tobacco smoking

(15)   Do you smoke?
         (Record 'yes' if regular smoker up to 1 month ago)   ☐

         If "no" to 15, ask:

(16)   Have you ever smoked?   ☐
         (Record 'no' if subject has never smoked as much as one cigarette a day, or
         30 g of tobacco a month, for as long as 1 year).
         Age when you stopped: ....

If "yes" to 15 or 16, fill in figures below:

	Amount smoked	
	Now	*Before stopping*
Cigarettes/day (average including weekends)	....	....
Grams of tobacco/week (hand-rolled cigarettes)	....	....
Grams of tobacco/week (pipe)	....	....
Cigars/week (large or small)	....	....

Occupation

(Record on dotted lines the number of years during which the subject has worked in any of these industries.)

(17) Have you ever worked in a dusty job?... ☐

(18) In a coal-mine .... ☐

(19) In any other mine .... ☐

(20) In a quarry .... ☐

(21) In a foundry .... ☐

(22) In a pottery .... ☐

(23) In a cotton, flax, or hemp mill .... ☐

(24) With asbestos .... ☐

(25) In any other dusty job .... ☐
       If "yes", specify ....
       ....

(26) Have you ever been exposed regularly to an irritating gas or to chemical fumes? ☐

       If "yes", give details of nature and duration:
       ....
       ....

Annex 2

Contributors and reviewers

LIST OF CONTRIBUTORS

A. Bergeret, Department of Occupational Medicine and Clinical Ergonomics, Jules Courmont Hospital, Centre Hospitalier Sud, Pierre Benite, France

T. Beritić, Institute for Medical Research and Occupational Health, Zagreb, Yugoslavia

M. G. Cassitto, Institute of Occupational Health, University of Milan, Milan, Italy

A. David, Medical Officer, Office of Occupational Health, World Health Organization, Geneva, Switzerland

B. D. Dinman, Aluminium Company of America, Pittsburg, USA

D. Djordjević, Consultant in Occupational Health, Pariske Komune, Belgrade, Yugoslavia

J. C. Duclos, Institute of Occupational Health, University of Lyons, Lyons, France

M. A. El Batawi, Chief Medical Officer, Office of Occupational Health, World Health Organization, Geneva, Switzerland

P. C. Elmes, Consultant in Occupational Health, Dawros House, St Andrew's Road, Dinas Powis, South Glamorgan, Wales

E. A. Emmett, Director, Division of Occupational Medicine, Johns Hopkins University, Baltimore, MD, USA

V. Foà, Institute of Occupational Health, University of Milan, Milan, Italy

R. Gilioli, Institute of Occupational Health, University of Milan, Milan, Italy

B. Gomboš, Department of Occupational Health, University Hospital, Košice, Czechoslovakia

J. M. Harrington, Institute of Occupational Health, University of Birmingham, England

C. H. Hine, Division of Occupational Medicine, University of California, San Francisco, CA, USA

J. V. Homewood, Cheshire, England

J. P. Hughes, Kaiser Aluminum and Chemical Corporation, Oakland, CA, USA

J. A. Indulski, Institute of Occupational Health, Łódź, Poland

L. Ivanova-Čemišanska, Institute of Hygiene and Occupational Health, Sofia, Bulgaria

J. Iżycki, Institute of Occupational Health, Łódź, Poland

L. Jirásek, Department of Dermatology, Medical School, Charles University, Prague, Czechoslovakia

E. P. Kindwall, Department of Hyperbaric Medicine, Milwaukee, USA

E. P. Krasnjuk, Research Institute of Labour Hygiene and Occupational Diseases, Kiev, Ukrainian Soviet Socialist Republic, USSR

J. Kuorinka, Institute of Occupational Health, Helsinki, Finland

K. Kurppa, Institute of Occupational Health, Helsinki, Finland

S. Langaard, Department of Occupational Medicine, Telemark Central Hospital, Grosgrun, Norway

R. Lauwerys, Department of Occupational and Clinical Toxicology, University of Louvain, Brussels, Belgium

L. P. Lubyanova, Research Institute of Labour Hygiene and Occupational Diseases, Kiev, Ukrainian Soviet Socialist Republic, USSR

A. D. McDonald, Research Institute for Occupational Health and Safety, Montreal, Canada

J. C. McDonald, Institute of Occupational Health and Safety, McGill University, Montreal, Canada

J. Merchant, National Institute for Occupational Safety and Health, Morgantown, WV, USA

A. M. Monaenkova, Institute of Labour Hygiene and Occupational Diseases, Moscow, USSR

L. S. Nikitina, Institute of Labour Hygiene and Occupational Diseases, Moscow, USSR

Z. Panova, Institute of Hygiene and Occupational Health, Sofia, Bulgaria

S. S. Pinto, Medical Department, ASARCO, Tacoma, WA, USA

I. Přerovská, Institute of Hygiene and Epidemiology, Centre of Industrial Hygiene and Occupational Diseases, Prague, Czechoslovakia

N. H. Proctor, Kaiser Aluminum and Chemical Corporation, Oakland, CA, USA

G. Prost, Institute of Occupational Health, University of Lyons, Lyons, France

M. Šarić, Institute for Medical Research and Occupational Health, Zagreb, Yugoslavia

V. Šedivec, Institute of Hygiene and Epidemiology, Centre of Industrial Hygiene and Occupational Diseases, Prague, Czechoslovakia

L. L. Sokolina, Institute of Labour Hygiene and Occupational Diseases, Moscow, USSR

H. Thiele, Central Institute for Occupational Health of the German Democratic Republic, Berlin, German Democratic Republic

M. Tolonen, Institute of Occupational Health, Helsinki, Finland

F. Tolot, Institute of Occupational Health, University of Lyons, Lyons, France

W. T. Ulmer, Research Institute for Silicosis, University of Bochum, Bochum Federal Republic of Germany

M. Vaněček, Institute of Hygiene and Epidemiology, Centre of Industrial Hygiene and Occupational Diseases, Prague, Czechoslovakia

A. E. Vermel, Institute of Labour Hygiene and Occupational Diseases, Moscow, USSR

K. S. Williamson, Imperial Chemical Industries, Alderley Works, Macclesfield, Cheshire, England

E. Zschunke, Central Institute for Occupational Health of the German Democratic Republic, Berlin, German Democratic Republic

WHO Scientific Group on Early Detection of Occupational Diseases

Geneva, 26 October to 1 November 1982

Members

S. E. Asogwa, Head, Department of Community Medicine, University of Nigeria, Enugu Campus, Enugu, Nigeria

A. Bergeret, Department of Occupational Medicine and Clinical Ergonomics, Jules Courmont Hospital, Centre Hospitalier Sud, Pierre Benite, France

D. Djordjević, Consultant in Occupational Health, Pariske Komune, Belgrade, Yugoslavia

P. C. Elmes, Consultant in Occupational Health, Dawros House, St Andrew's Road, Dinas Powis, South Glamorgan, Wales

E. A. Emmet, Director, Division of Occupational Medicine, School of Hygiene and Public Health, Johns Hopkins University, Baltimore, MD, USA (*Vice-Chairman*)

R. Gilioli, Institute of Occupational Health, University of Milan, Milan, Italy

Gu Xue-qi, Deputy Dean, School of Public Health, Shanghai First Medical College, Foon Lin Chiao, Shanghai, China

J. C. McDonald, Director, Institute of Occupational Health and Safety, McGill University, Montreal, Canada (*Rapporteur*)

A. O. Navakatikian, Deputy Director, Kiev Research Institute of Labour Hygiene and Occupational Diseases, Kiev, Ukrainian Soviet Socialist Republic, USSR

Y. Osman, Director, Occupational Health Department, Ministry of Health and Social Welfare, Khartoum, Sudan, (*Chairman*)

Secretariat

M. A. El Batawi, Chief Medical Officer, Office of Occupational Health, WHO, Geneva, Switzerland

A. David, Medical Officer, Office of Occupational Health, WHO Geneva, Switzerland (*Secretary*)

M. Nosál, Department of Occupational Health, University Hospital, Limbová, Bratislava-Kramár, Czechoslovakia (*Temporary Adviser*)[1]

Representative of International Labour Office

M. Stilon de Piro, Occupational Safety and Health Branch, ILO, Geneva, Switzerland

---

[1] Professor Nosál also represented the Permanent Commission and International Association on Occupational Health.

WHO publications may be obtained, direct or through booksellers, from:

ALGERIA: Entreprise nationale du Livre (ENAL), 3 bd Zirout Youcef, ALGIERS

ARGENTINA: Carlos Hirsch, SRL, Florida 165, Galerías Güemes, Escritorio 453/465, BUENOS AIRES

AUSTRALIA: Hunter Publications, 58A Gipps Street, COLLINGWOOD, VIC 3066 — Australian Government Publishing Service *(Mail order sales)*, P.O. Box 84, CANBERRA A.C.T. 2601; *or over the counter from:* Australian Government Publishing Service Booshops *at:* 70 Alinga Street, CANBERRA CITY A.C.T. 2600; 294 Adelaide Street, BRISBANE, Queensland 4000; 347 Swanston Street, MELBOURNE, VIC 3000; 309 Pitt Street, SYDNEY, N.S.W. 2000; Mt Newman House, 200 St. George's Terrace, PERTH, WA 6000; Industry House, 12 Pirie Street, ADELAIDE, SA 5000; 156–162 Macquarie Street, HOBART, TAS 7000 — R. Hill & Son Ltd., 608 St. Kilda Road, MELBOURNE, VIC 3004; Lawson House, 10–12 Clark Street, CROW'S NEST, NSW 2065

AUSTRIA: Gerold & Co., Graben 31, 1011 VIENNA I

BANGLADESH: The WHO Programme Coordinator, G.P.O Box 250, DHAKA 5

BELGIUM: *For books:* Office International de Librairie s.a., avenue Marnix 30, 1050 BRUSSELS. *For periodicals and subscriptions:* Office International des Périodiques, avenue Louise 485, 1050 BRUSSELS — *Subscriptions to World Health only:* Jean de Lannoy, 202 avenue du Roi, 1060 BRUSSELS

BHUTAN: *see* India, WHO Regional Office

BOTSWANA: Botsalo Books (Pty) Ltd., P.O. Box 1532, GABORONE

BRAZIL: Biblioteca Regional de Medicina OMS/OPS, Sector de Publicações, Caixa Postal 20.381, Vila Clementino, 04023 SÃO PAULO, S.P.

BURMA: *see* India, WHO Regional Office

CANADA: Canadian Public Health Association, 1335 Carling Avenue, Suite 210, OTTAWA, Ont. K1Z 8N8. (Tel: (613) 725–3769. Telex: 21–053–3841)

CHINA: China National Publications Import & Export Corporation, P.O. Box 88, BEIJING (PEKING)

DEMOCRATIC PEOPLE'S REPUBLIC OF KOREA: *see* India, WHO Regional Office

DENMARK: Munksgaard Export and Subscription Service, Nørre Søgade 35, 1370 COPENHAGEN K (Tel: + 45 1 12 85 70)

FIJI: The WHO Programme Coordinator, P.O. Box 113, SUVA

FINLAND: Akateeminen Kirjakauppa, Keskuskatu 2, 00101 HELSINKI 10

FRANCE: Librairie Arnette, 2 rue Casimir-Delavigne, 75006 PARIS

GERMAN DEMOCRATIC REPUBLIC: Buchhaus Leipzig, Postfach 140, 701 LEIPZIG

GERMANY FEDERAL REPUBLIC OF: Govi-Verlag GmbH, Ginnheimerstrasse 20, Postfach 5360, 6236 ESCHBORN — Buchhandlung Alexander Horn, Friedrichstrasse 39, Postfach 3340, 6200 WIESBADEN

GHANA: Fides Enterprises, P.O. Box 1628, ACCRA

GREECE: G.C. Eleftheroudakis S.A., Librairie internationale, rue Nikis 4, ATHENS (T. 126)

HONG KONG: Hong Kong Government Information Services, Beaconsfield House, 6th Floor, Queen's Road, Central, VICTORIA

HUNGARY: Kultura, P.O.B. 149, BUDAPEST 62

INDIA: WHO Regional Office for South-East Asia, World Health House, Indraprastha Estate, Mahatma Gandhi Road, NEW DELHI 110002

INDONESIA: P.T. Kalman Media Pusaka, Pusat Perdagangan Senen, Block 1, 4th Floor, P.O. Box 3433/Jkt, JAKARTA

IRAN (ISLAMIC REPUBLIC OF): Iran University Press, 85 Park Avenue, P.O. Box 54/551, TEHERAN

IRELAND: TDC Publishers, 12 North Frederick Street, DUBLIN 1 (Tel: 744835–749677)

ISRAEL: Heiliger & Co., 3 Nathan Strauss Street, JERUSALEM 94227

ITALY: Edizioni Minerva Medica, Corso Bramante 83–85, 10126 TURIN; Via Lamarmora 3, 20100 MILAN; Via Spallanzani 9, 00161 ROME

JAPAN: Maruzen Co. Ltd., P.O. Box 5050, TOKYO International, 100–31

JORDAN: Jordan Book Centre Co. Ltd., University Street, P.O. Box 301 (Al-Jubeiha), AMMAN

KUWAIT: The Kuwait Bookshops Co. Ltd., Thunayan Al-Ghanem Bldg, P.O. Box 2942, KUWAIT

LAOS PEOPLE'S DEMOCRATIC REPUBLIC: The WHO Programme Coordinator, P.O. Box 343, VIENTIANE

LUXEMBOURG: Librairie du Centre, 49 bd Royal, LUXEMBOURG

MALAWI: Malawi Book Service, P.O. Box 30044, Chichiti, BLANTYRE 3

WHO publications may be obtained, direct or through booksellers, from:

MALAYSIA: The WHO Programme Coordinator, Room 1004, 10th Floor, Wisma Lim Foo Yong (formerly Fitzpatrick's Building), Jalan Raja Chulan, KUALA LUMPUR 05-10; P.O. Box 2550, KUALA LUMPUR 01-02; Parry's Book Center, 124-1 Jalan Tun Sambanthan, P.O. Box 10960, 50730 KUALA LUMPUR

MALDIVES: *See* India, WHO Regional Office

MEXICO: Librería Internacional, S.A. de C.V., Av. Sonora 206, 06100-MÉXICO, D.F.

MONGOLIA: *see* India, WHO Regional Office

MOROCCO: Editions La Porte, 281 avenue Mohammed V, RABAT

NEPAL: *see* India, WHO Regional Office

NETHERLANDS: Medical Books Europe BV, Noorderwal 38, 7241 BL LOCHEM

NEW ZEALAND: New Zealand Government Printing Office, Publishing Administration, Private Bag, WELLINGTON; Walter Street, WELLINGTON; World Trade Building, Cubacade, Cuba Street, WELLINGTON, *Government Bookshops at:* Hannaford Burton Building, Rutland Street, Private Bag, AUCKLAND; 159 Hereford Street, Private Bag, CHRISTCHURCH; Alexandra Street, P.O. Box 857, HAMILTON; T & G Building, Princes Street, P.O. Box 1104, DUNEDIN — R. Hill & Son Ltd, Ideal House, Cnr Gillies Avenue & Eden Street, Newmarket, AUCKLAND 1

NORWAY: Tanum — Karl Johan A.S., P.O. Box 1177, Sentrum, N-0107 OSLO 1

PAKISTAN: Mirza Book Agency, 65 Shahrah-E-Quaid-E-Azam, P.O. Box 729, LAHORE 3

PAPUA NEW GUINEA: The WHO Programme Coordinator, P.O. Box 646, KONEDOBU

PHILIPPINES: World Health Organization, Regional Office for the Western Pacific, P.O. Box 2932, MANILA

PORTUGAL: Livraria Rodrigues, 186 Rua do Ouro, LISBON 2

REPUBLIC OF KOREA: The WHO Programme Coordinator, Central P.O. Box 540, SEOUL

SINGAPORE: The WHO Programme Coordinator, 144 Moulmein Road, SINGAPORE 1130; Newton P.O. Box 31, SINGAPORE 9122

SOUTH AFRICA: *Contact major book stores*

SPAIN: Ministerio de Sanidad y Consumo, Centro de publicaciones, Documentación y Biblioteca, Paseo del Prado 18, 28014 MADRID — Comercial Atheneum S.A., Consejo de Ciento 130-136, 08015 BARCELONA; General Moscardó 29, MADRID 20 — Librería Díaz de Santos, P.O. Box 6050, 28006 MADRID; Balmes 417 y 419, 08022 BARCELONA

SRI LANKA: *see* India, WHO Regional Office

SWEDEN: *For books:* Aktiebolaget C.E. Fritzes Kungl. Hovbokhandel, Regeringsgatan 12, 103 27 STOCKHOLM. *For periodicals:* Wennergren-Williams AB, Box 30004, 104 25 STOCKHOLM

SWITZERLAND: Medizinischer Verlag Hans Huber, Länggassstrasse 76, 3012 BERN 9

THAILAND: *see* India, WHO Regional Office

UNITED KINGDOM: H.M. Stationery Office: 49 High Holborn, LONDON WC1V 6HB; 13a Castle Street, EDINBURGH EH2 3AR, 80 Chichester Street, BELFAST BT1 4JY; Brazennose Street, MANCHESTER M60 8AS; 258 Broad Street, BIRMINGHAM B1 2HE; Southey House, Wine Street, BRISTOL BS1 2BQ. *All mail orders should be sent to:* HMSO Publications Centre, 51 Nine Elms Lane, LONDON SW8 5DR

UNITED STATES OF AMERICA: *Copies of individual publications (not subscriptions):* WHO Publications Center USA, 49 Sheridan Avenue, ALBANY, NY 12210. *Subscription orders and correspondence concerning subscriptions should be addressed to the* World Health Organization, Distribution and Sales, 1211 GENEVA 27, Switzerland. *Publications are also available from the* United Nations Bookshop, NEW YORK, NY 10017 *(retail only)*

USSR: *For readers in the USSR requiring Russian editions:* Komsomolskij prospekt 18, Medicinskaja Kniga, MOSCOW — *For readers outside the USSR requiring Russian editions:* Kuzneckij most 18, Meždunarodnaja Kniga, MOSCOW G-200

VENEZUELA: Librería Medica Paris, Apartado 60.681, CARACAS 106

YUGOSLAVIA: Jugoslovenska Knjiga, Terazije 27/II, 11000 BELGRADE

Special terms for developing countries are obtainable on application to the WHO Programme Coordinators or WHO Regional Offices listed above or to the World Health Organization, Distribution and Sales Service, 1211 Geneva 27, Switzerland. Orders from countries where sales agents have not yet been appointed may also be sent to the Geneva address, but must be paid for in pounds sterling, US dollars, or Swiss francs. Unesco book coupons may also be used.

Prices are subject to change without notice.